Department of Health
Welsh Office
Scottish Home and Health Department
Department of Health and Social Security, Northern Ireland

Report on Confidential Enquiries into Maternal Deaths in the United Kingdom 1985-87

London: HMSO

ISBN 0 11 321333 6

CONTENTS

PREFACE

United Kingdom Confidential Enquiries Into Maternal Deaths Report 1985–87

This is the first report on confidential enquiries into maternal deaths combining information from the four countries of the United Kingdom (UK). This and preceding reports from England and Wales, Scotland, and Northern Ireland represent the longest running series of continuous clinical audit in the world.

The report replaces three separate reports, those for England and Wales, Scotland, and Northern Ireland. The England and Wales reports were published three-yearly from 1952–54 to 1982–84. The reports for Scotland were published at different intervals from 1965–71 to 1981–85, the latest covering both maternal and perinatal deaths; however future issues in the Scottish series will, for maternal deaths, include statistical data only. The reports for Northern Ireland were started in 1956 and were published four-yearly until 1967; because of the small number of maternal deaths the next report covered the ten year period from 1968–77, and the last report the seven year period 1978–84.

The decision to change to a combined UK report on maternal deaths was made by the four Chief Medical Officers in 1984 with the encouragement and on the recommendation of the Royal College of Obstetricians and Gynaecologists. Apart from the obvious advantages of looking at maternal mortality from a UK perspective, a problem had arisen for the enquiries in Scotland and to an even greater extent in Northern Ireland due to the relatively small number of deaths which had occurred in recent years. While this reduction in mortality was obviously satisfactory, it did mean that there was considerable difficulty for the authors of these reports in describing and discussing illustrative cases, while at the same time maintaining the necessary confidentiality. Assessing the cases from the four countries together has helped to solve the problem while making fuller use of the information available.

This report covers a total of 265 cases which were reported to the enquiry, 212 for England, 18 from Wales, 25 from Scotland and 10 from Northern Ireland. Only 16 of these were Late deaths (ie those occurring more than 42 days after pregnancy and delivery), in contrast to 73 Late deaths reported to the last England and Wales enquiry in 1982–84. This reduction is the result of a policy decision by the English and Welsh Assessors not to continue to collect information on these cases routinely. The reasons for this decision are fully discussed in the separate chapter on 'Late deaths', Chapter 15, to which they have been assigned.

When the 16 Late deaths had been excluded, the remaining 249 deaths were 139 Direct Obstetric deaths (56%), 84 Indirect Obstetric deaths (34%) and 26 Fortuitous deaths (10%) (ie considered to be unrelated to the pregnancy). The 139 Direct deaths for this triennium compare with 163 for the UK in 1982–84. The report includes details of all but one of the known Direct obstetric deaths. This followed a termination of pregnancy and was reported to the enquiry, but information was not made available for assessment as the case is the subject of legal proceedings.

The 22 Indirect deaths and one Direct death which were related to cardiac disease are described in Chapter 11, and the remaining 62 Indirect deaths are described in Chapter 12. The Fortuitous deaths are listed in Chapter 14.

The authors have taken the opportunity provided by the introduction of what is expected to be a new series of reports to make some changes in the content and order of the chapters. However, as it was also appreciated that many readers of the report are interested in the trends in different causes of death through a time series, the statisticians have in many of the tables separated out figures relating to England and Wales for 1985–87 for comparison with previous reports, as well as giving UK figures. These changes are more fully explained in the Foreword (Page ix).

In view of the very small number of deaths following spontaneous or legal abortion, and the absence of any maternal death due to criminal abortion, it was decided to discontinue the individual chapter on abortion, and include these deaths with other 'Early pregnancy deaths' in Chapter 6. Another change is that deaths from pulmonary embolism are now included with other deaths from thromboembolism in Chapter 4.

The commonest causes of maternal death were thromboembolism and hypertensive disorders of pregnancy. Compared with previous reports for England and Wales, a higher proportion of deaths from thromboembolism, more than half, occurred in the antenatal period, and in many cases the diagnosis did not appear even to have been considered.

Although the death rate from hypertensive disorders of pregnancy was similar to the rate previously reported from England and Wales, there was an unexpected change in the immediate cause of death. In the England and Wales report for 1982–84, 21 of the 25 cases had cerebral complications, whereas in the present triennium there was a shift to deaths from respiratory complications and nine of the 26 cases died from the adult respiratory distress syndrome (ARDS). It appeared that some of the patients were surviving the initial period, when they had previously been at greatest risk from inadequately controlled hypertension causing cerebral haemorrhage, only to die later from progressive ARDS despite mechanical ventilation and intensive care.

In this triennium deaths related to cardiac disease were the third commonest cause of death. The last Scottish report (1981–85) had already noted an increase in deaths from this cause, but it had not been observed in England and Wales. These were mainly Indirect deaths. There appeared to be a newly identifiable group of patients with congenital heart disease, who had been treated apparently successfully by surgery, but who were then unable to cope with the additional circulatory load of pregnancy and labour. These women, who sometimes become pregnant against advice and continue with the pregnancy, need particularly careful monitoring throughout pregnancy and labour, and after delivery. They require expert attention from teams of obstetricians, cardiologists and anaesthetists, and delivery in a unit with proper facilities to deal with their special problems.

The number of deaths from ectopic pregnancy and the rate per million estimated pregnancies for England and Wales remained unchanged since 1982–84. Unfortunately the rate for the UK cannot be calculated as the number of pregnancies cannot be estimated from the data available (see Chapter 1), nor are there data for 1985–87 for the number of women with ectopic pregnancy admitted to hospital. However it is hoped that improved methods of early diagnosis for the condition will produce a reduction in the number of deaths in the future and that death rates will be available for the next report.

There was a definite reduction in the number of deaths judged to be directly attributable to anaesthesia compared with the last report for England and Wales. However there was also a larger number of cases in which the anaesthesia was considered to have contributed to the death. This in part reflects a change in the perception of the anaesthetists' role and responsibilities in the management of obstetric cases. They need to be involved from an early stage in the monitoring and management of high risk patients, such as those with severe pre-eclampsia, even if operative delivery is not planned. It is recommended that expert assistance should always be available to all anaesthetists and that centralised recovery and high dependency care facilities should be provided in maternity units.

There were ten deaths directly due to antepartum and postpartum haemorrhage but in considerably more cases blood loss was an additional factor. The authors have again included suggested guidelines for an agreed procedure for the management of massive haemorrhage in obstetric units. These, somewhat modified from the last 1982–84 England and Wales report, are detailed in the Annexe to Chapter 3.

The number of deaths from genital sepsis remained low but the need for early accurate bacteriological diagnosis and treatment with appropriate antibiotics is stressed. An effective treatment for amniotic fluid embolism has not yet been identified.

Unfortunately it was not possible to calculate a rate for deaths following Caesarean section in the UK as denominator data were not available. There was a small decline in the total number of deaths for England and Wales since the last report. However an unacceptably high proportion of deaths of women delivered by Caesarean section continued to be associated with substandard care. Greater supervision of junior staff and improved facilities for resuscitation are recommended.

The 84 Indirect deaths accounted for 38% of the Direct and Indirect cases included in the Enquiry. The largest group was 16 deaths from intracranial haemorrhage, unrelated to the hypertensive disorders of pregnancy. Some of them were identified at autopsy as being due to rupture of a 'berry aneurysm', but in many cases the source of bleeding was not identified.

In Chapter 16 the emphasis is put on the need for better communication between all those concerned in the clinical care of the patients and the pathologists investigating the cause of death. An autopsy should always be performed for a maternal death. To improve the standard of the autopsies greater use should be made in England of the expert panels of pathologists available in each region in close liaison with the Regional Pathology Assessor. It is a matter of concern that histological examination was not performed in a large proportion of maternal deaths referred to coroners and procurators fiscal.

In Chapter 17 the authors have highlighted the principal lessons learnt from a review of the major causes of maternal death, and have made recommendations for improvements in clinical care and provision of facilities in the maternity services. The continued downward trend in maternal mortality in this triennium from 163 Direct obstetric deaths in 1982–84 for the United Kingdom to 139 must be regarded as evidence of improved maternity care. However the fact that the assessors considered that substandard care was present in the majority of Direct deaths indicates that it should be possible to achieve a further reduction.

It was apparent from the detailed analysis of maternal deaths that in many instances they reflect deficiencies in the maternity services available. Failure of communication of potential problems to more senior and experienced midwives, doctors, obstetricians or anaesthetists was often noted and frequently these features were due to the splitting of obstetric and gynaecological services on more than one site. A reappraisal of the total staff, midwifery and medical, available to provide adequate cover on a 24-hour basis is required by all obstetric units and there should be a regular review of this service available. The necessity to avoid split sites and to provide comprehensive cover should be taken into account in any new arrangements proposed for obstetric services under the new NHS and Community Services Act.

We wish to thank and acknowledge the work of the Editorial Board which was formed from Assessors from each country to decide the main issues of policy and administration for the report. They met first under the Chairmanship of Dr Michael Abrams and later of Dr Jeremy Metters (Deputy Chief Medical Officers of the Department of Health). The members of the Editorial Board (listed at the beginning of the report) were the National Assessors for England, Wales and Northern Ireland and representative Assessors from the Scottish confidential enquiry, supported by statisticians, and four senior Departmental medical staff. The Assessors formed the clinical sub-group, under the chairmanship of Professor V R Tindall, and were responsible for the writing of the chapters, either individually, or in small partnerships and produced the first drafts for general consideration. The statisticians were co-ordinated by Mrs Beverley Botting of the Medical Statistics Unit of the Office of Population Censuses and Surveys, who also prepared the Introduction (Chapter 1). Together they have produced the report and overcome, by careful co-ordination, the considerable logistical problems of the combination of information from the four countries.

We should like to thank all those who contributed to the individual case reports in England, Wales, Scotland and Northern Ireland. These include the obstetricians, anaesthetists, pathologists, District Medical Officers (DMOs), consultants in public health medicine, Chief Administrative Medical Officers (CAMOs), general practitioners and midwives, and also the coroners and procurators fiscal, who made their reports available to the enquiry. We are most grateful to all the Assessors in the four countries who have given generously of their time and expertise in the assessment of cases. They have also provided comments on the contents of the chapters of the report. The final assessment and recommendations take into account the views expressed by all the Assessors which were co-ordinated by the authors to produce a report generally acceptable to all who contributed.

We consider that the first combined UK report of the confidential enquiries into maternal deaths has made a most satisfactory and encouraging start. It is expected to be the first of an invaluable series, whose aim is to reduce maternal mortality further, and for this purpose we endorse the recommendations made in Chapter 17.

CMO England Donald Acheson

CMO Scotland Kenneth Calman

CMO Wales Deirdre Hine

CMO N Ireland James McKenna

FOREWORD

It was decided that for this triennium, 1985–87, maternal deaths for the whole of the United Kingdom* (UK) would be considered, and that some changes would be made in the format of the report, compared with those for England and Wales, for Scotland and for Northern Ireland up to 1984. Unless otherwise specified, changes described are from previous England and Wales reports. Difficulties with obtaining some statistical information have resulted in changes and omissions in some of the tables.

The content and order of the Report

The Introduction, Chapter 1, includes recent trends in fertility and non-clinical aspects of maternal deaths. It also provides a statistical background and overview to the rest of the chapters. Chapters 2 to 10 deal with Direct obstetric deaths; Chapter 11 covers Cardiac disease with both Direct and Indirect deaths, and Chapter 12 other Indirect deaths; Chapter 13 deals with Caesarean section; Chapters 14 and 15 with Fortuitous and Late deaths; Chapter 16 with pathology; and Chapter 17 with general and specific Recommendations derived from the other chapters. There is no longer a separate chapter on abortion and these cases are now included in Chapter 6 (Early pregnancy deaths).

The title of Chapter 2 has been changed from 'Hypertensive diseases' to 'Hypertensive disorders of pregnancy' in line with recent practice. Chapter 3 is titled 'Antepartum and postpartum haemorrhage' to clarify the fact that only these particular types of uterine haemorrhage are included. Chapter 4 has been titled 'Thrombosis and thromboembolism' to include cases of thrombosis as well as pulmonary embolism. Chapter 6, titled 'Early pregnancy deaths (including abortion)', contains deaths from ectopic pregnancy and all types of abortion. Chapter 8, titled 'Genital tract trauma', includes cases of ruptured uterus and damage to the cervix. Chapter 12, titled 'Other Indirect deaths', illustrates the fact that some Indirect deaths are also included in Chapter 11, 'Cardiac disease associated with pregnancy'.

Changes in statistical tables

1. The previous triennial reports were concerned with maternal deaths in England and Wales. Scotland and Northern Ireland published their own reports. The current report for 1985–87 includes all component countries of the UK. To enable comparison with previous data for England and Wales, 1985–87 data for England and Wales are also usually presented

---

* References to the United Kingdom include all four countries; those referring to Great Britain exclude Northern Ireland.

separately. We plan to include a similar dual presentation of data for the next report based on 1988–90 maternal deaths, but the following report (dealing with 1991–93) will not include any England and Wales comparisons since we will then have three triennia of UK data. Basic statistical tables for Scotland will be published in the quinquennial series of reports on maternal and perinatal deaths in Scotland.

2. The collection of hospital inpatient statistics ended after 1985 in England and Wales and was not replaced until 1987 by new hospital episode statistics. Unfortunately at the time of writing these new data were not available. In contrast Wales continued to collect HAA statistics. As a result no data on spontaneous abortions or ectopic pregnancies are available for inclusion in the denominator data for calculating rates. There are also no data on the number of Caesarean sections performed.

3. Tables showing the data presented by parity have been dropped from individual cause of death chapters (such as 'Hypertensive disorders of pregnancy'). This is because at birth, registration information is only collected for births within marriage. Over a quarter of all children are now born outside marriage and so for these births there is no parity information collected. Because of the interrelationship between parity and age, and in view of the small numbers of maternal deaths for a given condition when subdivided into parity, it was decided that such data are increasingly difficult to analyse, and they have therefore been omitted. Also no data on the country-of-birth of the mother can be published as this is not available from the confidential enquiry forms.

Substandard care

The term substandard care has been used in this report to take into account not only failure in clinical care, but also some of the underlying factors which may have produced a low standard of care for the patient. This includes situations produced by the action of the woman herself, or her relatives, which may be outside the control of the clinicians. It also takes into account shortage of resources for staffing facilities; and administrative failure in the maternity services and the back-up facilities such as anaesthetic, radiological and pathology services. It is used in preference to the term 'avoidable factors' which was used previously in the England and Wales reports until 1979 and has also been used in all the separate Scottish and Northern Ireland reports. This was sometimes misinterpreted in the past, and taken to mean that avoiding these factors would necessarily have prevented the death. 'Substandard' in the context of the report means that the care that the patient received, or the care that was made available to her, fell below the standard which the authors considered should have been offered to her in this triennium.

CHAPTER 1

Introduction

Trends in maternal mortality

Scotland and Northern Ireland have now joined with England and Wales to combine data on maternal mortality, so for the first time this report covers maternal deaths in the United Kingdom (UK). Previous reports have been concerned with maternal deaths in England and Wales, in Scotland and in Northern Ireland separately.

The report is based on individual case reports. Information was collected from all the professionals who had been concerned with the care of the women, and whose case reports were then passed to Regional and National Assessors. Strict confidentiality is observed at all stages of the enquiry.

This chapter presents statistics which provide a background to maternal deaths described elsewhere in this report. Tables 1.1 to 1.4 present data drawn exclusively from other official sources and not from the enquiry.

During the 36 years of these enquiries more than 30 million births have been registered in the UK. Figure 1.1 shows the general fertility rate (births per 1,000 women aged 15–44 years) over this period, and combined data for each triennium are given in Table 1.1. The figure shows increasing fertility between 1952 and 1964 followed by steadily decreasing rates until 1977. The rate then fluctuated, but since 1982 there has been a small but sustained increase. Table 1.1 shows that both the number of births and the birth rate in 1985–87 were slightly higher than those experienced in the previous triennium.

Table 1.1 *Total number of births (live and still), United Kingdom, 1952–87.*

Year of occurrence	Total births (in thousands)	Rate per 1000 women aged 15–44 years
1952–54*	2,446.6	78.2
1955–57*	2,521.8	82.6
1958–60*	2,722.2	90.0
1961–63	2,964.7	93.5
1964–66	3,040.4	94.0
1967–69	2,870.2	89.3
1970–72	2,673.4	83.2
1973–75	2,239.2	68.8
1976–78	2,038.3	60.9
1979–81	2,235.4	64.2
1982–84	2,183.2	60.7
1985–87	2,293.5	61.9

* 1952–60 data exclude Northern Ireland.
Source: England & Wales — Birth statistics
Series FM1 No. 11 Table 3.2; FM1 No. 13 Table 1.1, 1.2; FM1 No. 16 Table 1.1, 1.2
Scotland — Registrar General's Annual Report 1988 Table A 1.3
Northern Ireland — Registrar General's Annual Report 1987 Table E1.

Figure 1.1 General fertility rate, United Kingdom 1952–87

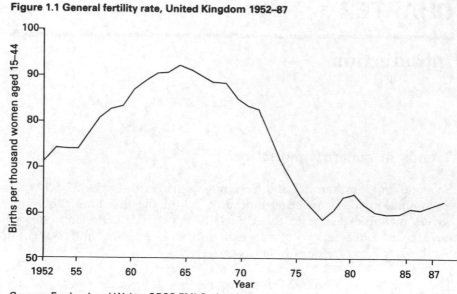

Source: England and Wales: OPCS FMI Series data
Scotland: Registrar General, Annual Report, Scotland
Northern Ireland: Registrar General, Annual Report, Northern Ireland

Figure 1.2 Legal Abortion Rate, Great Britain 1970–87

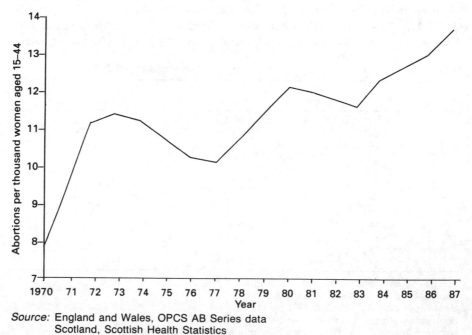

Source: England and Wales, OPCS AB Series data
Scotland, Scottish Health Statistics

There has been a steady reduction in maternal mortality over the past 30 years. The confidential enquiry includes deaths of women after legal or spontaneous abortion and some of the reduction in maternal mortality since 1970 reflects the introduction of legal abortion. The initial introduction of legal abortion is said to reduce and in the longer term eliminate mortality after illegal abortion[1]. Since 1970 there has been a consistent decline in deaths from illegal abortion. In 1970–72 there were 37 deaths from illegal abortion; in 1979–81 there was one; and in the more recent triennia there have been none. Between the implementation of the Abortion Acts in 1968 in England and Wales and in Scotland, and the end of 1987, over 2 million legal terminations of pregnancy were carried out on residents of Great Britain. In Northern Ireland only a small number of terminations is done on medical grounds under the case law which applied in England, Wales and Scotland before the 1967 Abortion Act. Some women having terminations in Great Britain, however, give their usual address as being in Northern Ireland. This was the case for 5,112 terminations in Great Britain between 1985 and 1987.

Table 1.2 shows both the number of terminations and the rate per 1,000 women aged 15–44 years for each triennium since the introduction of legal abortion. Figure 1.2 shows the legal abortion rate for each individual year over the same period. Whilst the rate has both risen and fallen from year to year, there appears to be an overall upward trend. During 1985–87 there were just over 475,000 terminations to women resident in Great Britain, an increase of 13% compared with the previous triennium. However, since the number of women aged 15–44 years also rose between 1982–84 and 1985–87, in 1985–87 the abortion rate per 1,000 women aged 15–44 years was 13.2, 10% higher than in 1982–84.

Table 1.2 *Legal abortions to women resident in Great Britain, 1970–87.*

Triennium	No. of Abortions	Rate per 1,000 women aged 15–44 years
1970–72	299,529	9.6
1973–75	351,856	11.1
1976–78	341,191	10.5
1979–81	406,133	12.0
1982–84	420,876	12.0
1985–87	475,330	13.2

Source: England and Wales: Abortion Statistics,
                        Series AB No 14 Table 2
        Scotland: Scottish Health Statistics,
                        1987, 88 Table 5.3

Table 1.3 presents some statistics of maternal mortality and births in the UK from the Registrars General for every third triennium between 1955–57 and 1982–84 and for 1985–87. Over this period the maternal mortality rate, expressed per 100,000 total births, fell from 67.1 to 7.6. This represents a reduction of approximately 20% per triennium assuming a constant rate of fall. Between 1982–84 and 1985–87 the maternal mortality rate fell by 18%, maintaining this rate of decrease.

3

Table 1.3 *Some statistics of maternal mortality and births, United Kingdom 1955–87.*

	1955–57†	1964–66‡	1973–75*	1982–84**	1985–87**
Total maternal deaths	1,691	1,011	408	203	174
Total births	2,521,804	3,040,378	2,239,233	2,183,151	2,293,508
Maternal mortality rate per 100,000 total births	67.1	33.3	18.2	9.3	7.6
General fertility rate per 1,000 women aged 15–44 years	83	94	69	61	62

† ICD 6th Revision: ICD 650–652, 640–649, 660–689
‡ ICD 7th Revision: ICD 650–652, 640–649, 660–689
* ICD 8th Revision: ICD 640–645, 630–639, 650–678
** ICD 9th Revision: ICD 630–639, 640–676
Figures from Registrars General:
1955–57 Great Britain only as stillbirths not available prior to 1961 for Northern Ireland.
Source: England & Wales — 1955–75 Mortality statistics, childhood and maternity,
Series DH3 No. 4 Table 18.
1982–86 Mortality statistics, cause, Series DH2, Table 2.
1987 End of year cause computer run.
1955–83 Birth statistics, Series FM1, No. 11, Table 1.1, 1.2.
1984–87 Birth statistics, Series FM1, No 16, Table 1.1, 1.2.
Scotland — 1987 Annual Report of Registrar General
Northern Ireland — 1987 Annual Report of Registrar General

To place these maternal mortality rates in context, it has been estimated elsewhere[2] that maternal deaths per thousand births are 6.4 in Africa, 4.2 in Asia, and 2.7 in Latin America, compared with 0.3 in all developed countries and less than 0.1 in Northern and Middle Europe. This is consistent with the current rate of 0.07 in the UK.

Maternal deaths can also be expressed per 1,000 women aged 15–44 years. Maternal mortality rates calculated in this way (Table 1.4) have fallen faster than the death rates from all causes for women in the same age-group. Between 1961–63, the first triennium for which data are available for the whole UK, and 1985–87 the mortality rate for women aged 15–44 years fell by 38% from 1,006.8 deaths per million women to 622.5, whereas over the same period the maternal mortality rate fell by 86% from 29.7 to 4.2; in 1985–87 maternal deaths comprised less than 1% of all deaths of women in this age-group, compared with 3% in 1961–63.

The 1985–87 enquiry

Maternal deaths are subclassified into 'Direct' deaths resulting from obstetric complications of pregnancy, labour and the puerperium; 'Indirect' deaths resulting from either a previous existing disease, or from a disease which developed during pregnancy, and which was aggravated by pregnancy; and 'Fortuitous' deaths resulting from causes not related to or influenced by pregnancy.

Figure 1.3 Maternal deaths, United Kingdom 1985–87

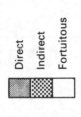

Direct
Indirect
Fortuitous

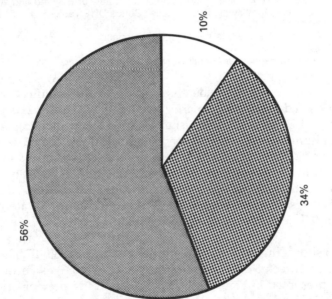

56%

10%

34%

Source: Confidential enquiries into maternal deaths

Table 1.4 *Mortality rates per million population aged 15–44 years; All causes and maternal deaths, United Kingdom 1952–87.*

Triennium	Mortality rates per million females aged 15–44 years		
	All causes	Maternal deaths	% of deaths in the age-group that are due to maternal causes
1952–54*	1,354.2	54.1	4.0
1955–57*	1,184.2	41.7	3.5
1958–60*	1,069.7	35.5	3.3
1961–63	1,006.8	29.7	3.0
1964–66	966.1	23.8	2.5
1967–69	893.2	18.0	2.0
1970–72	847.0	13.7	1.6
1973–75	807.9	9.0	1.1
1976–78	763.2	7.5	1.0
1979–81	697.2	6.6	1.0
1982–84	641.7	4.7	0.7
1985–87	622.5	4.2	0.7

* 1952–60 data are for Great Britain only.
ICD 6th revision: 1952–57, ICD 640–689
ICD 7th revision: 1958–67, ICD 640–689
ICD 8th revision: 1968–77, ICD 630–678
ICD 9th revision: 1978–87, ICD 630–676
Sources: England and Wales
        1952–73 Registrar General's statistical review of England and Wales, Part I.
        1974–87 Mortality statistics, cause. Series DH2 Table 2.
    Scotland
        Registrar General's Annual Report, Scotland.
    Northern Ireland
        Registrar General's Annual Report, Northern Ireland.

In 1985–87 there were 265 deaths known to the enquiry, of which 249 (94%) occurred during pregnancy or before 42 days postpartum (the International Definition of Maternal Death). The remaining 16 deaths for this triennium are classed as 'Late' deaths and are considered separately in Chapter 15. The total number of maternal deaths reported to the enquiry is consistent with a continued reduction in maternal mortality. UK data for the previous triennia are not available, but the 216 maternal deaths during 1985–87 of residents of England and Wales (excluding Late deaths) represents a fall of 11% compared with 1982–84.

Table 1.5 shows that of the 249 maternal deaths in 1985–87 139 (56%) were classified as Direct, 84 (34%) as Indirect, and 26 (10%) as Fortuitous. These data are presented in Figure 1.3. Data given in the previous report (based on only England and Wales data) showed a similar distribution (57% Direct, 29% Indirect and 14% Fortuitous).

Table 1.5 also shows that 74 women (30%) died before the twenty-eighth week of pregnancy; a similar proportion of early maternal deaths as in England and Wales data for the previous triennium (29%). Five maternal deaths before 28 weeks gestation were associated with a live birth.

The wide regional variation in maternal mortality is shown in Table 1.6. The period 1976–87 is used to increase the number of maternal deaths in the UK available for analysis. Rates for 1976–87 for the UK constituent countries showed the highest Direct obstetric maternal mortality rate to be

Table 1.5 *Reported deaths in relation to stage of pregnancy at which death occurred: United Kingdom 1985–87*

	Direct deaths	Indirect deaths	Fortuitous deaths	Total
Total (excluding Late deaths)	139	84	26	249
Deaths under 28 weeks gestation	43	23	8	74
of which: After abortion	7	8	2	17
Ectopic pregnancy	14	—	—	14
Undelivered	18	14	6	38
Delivery of liveborn	4	1	—	5
Deaths from 28 weeks gestation to 6 weeks postpartum	96	61	18	175
of which: Undelivered	14	12	7	33
Delivered	82	49	11	142
Deaths later than 6 weeks postpartum	6	8	2	16

in Scotland (8.9 per 100,000 total births) and the lowest to be in Wales (7.2). In the Regional Health Authorities (RHAs) of England over this period the Direct obstetric maternal mortality rate per 100,000 total births varied between 10.6 per 100,000 births in East Anglian RHA and 5.8 per 100,000 births in South West Thames RHA. This variation was, however, smaller than that given in a similar analysis based on 1976–84 given in the previous report where the rates varied between 6.1 and 12.4 per 100,000 births. Overall between 1976 and 1987 in the RHAs of England the ratio for Direct to Indirect deaths was approximately 2:1 but this ratio varied considerably at regional level.

Table 1.6 *Reported Direct and Indirect maternal mortality by area of residence, 1976–87*

Area of residence	Reported			Direct obstetric mortality rate**	Perinatal mortality rate†
	Total births	Direct deaths*	Indirect deaths		
United Kingdom	8,744,423	744	359‡	8.5	12.5
England	7,186,599	613	285	8.5	12.3
Wales	429,567	31	27	7.2	13.1
Scotland	797,917	71	45	8.9	12.7
Northern Ireland* **	330,340	29	2‡	8.8	14.6
Regional Health Authorities					
Northern	476,492	50	20	10.5	13.4
Yorkshire	557,033	42	31	7.5	13.6
Trent	691,958	60	32	8.7	12.5
East Anglian	284,020	30	14	10.6	10.7
North West Thames	554,279	47	14	8.5	11.1
North East Thames	603,427	62	11	10.3	12.0
South East Thames	537,797	39	17	7.2	12.0
South West Thames	416,712	24	15	5.8	10.9
Wessex	401,735	25	12	6.2	11.0
Oxford	379,918	24	14	6.3	10.6
South Western	444,342	29	21	6.5	11.4
West Midlands	818,720	85	31	10.4	14.3
Mersey	380,414	35	22	9.2	12.6
North Western	639,752	61	31	9.4	13.4

*   Includes abortion.
** Per 100,000 total births.
†   Stillbirths & deaths under 1 week combined per 1,000 live and stillbirths.
‡   85–87 data only.

Table 1.6 also shows the perinatal mortality rates for the UK, and for each constituent country and RHA of England over the same period. These rates, together with the maternal mortality rates are shown in Figure 1.4a and 1.4b, the RHAs in England ordered by decreasing maternal mortality rates. Whilst Northern and West Midlands RHAs had among the highest rates for both direct obstetric mortality and perinatal mortality, and South West Thames, Oxford and Wessex RHAs had among the lowest rates for both categories, some other regions showed a less consistent pattern. Kendall's rank correlation test based upon the ranked order of the Direct obstetric mortality rate and that of the perinatal mortality for Scotland, Wales, Northern Ireland and the RHAs of England showed a statistically significant association at the 5% level (one tail test).

Pregnancies

In accordance with established custom in the reports for England and Wales, in most of the succeeding chapters of this report maternal deaths will be related to the number of maternities (mothers delivered of live or stillborn infants) rather than to the total number of births, since this latter statistic is slightly inflated by multiple births. In England and Wales the combination of the numbers of maternities, together with terminations, adjusted to allow for the period of gestation, provide data which are referred to in official statistics as 'conceptions'. These statistics are based on the estimated date of conception. This explains the differences between these data and those given in previous tables in this chapter which are based on the date of delivery. These data are not available for Scotland and Northern Ireland.

In Table 1.7 an estimate has been made of the number of 'pregnancies' in England and Wales. For all triennia before 1985 the number of hospital admissions for spontaneous abortions (at less than 28 weeks' gestation) and ectopic pregnancies have been added to the official 'conception' statistics. This total is clearly an underestimate of the actual number of pregnancies since not all women whose pregnancy ends in spontaneous abortion are admitted to hospital. Whilst Wales has continued to collect HAA statistics, the collection of hospital inpatient statistics ended in England after 1985 to be replaced for 1987 onwards by new hospital episode statistics. Unfortunately at the time of writing these data were not available. Therefore an estimate of the number of hospital admissions has been made based on the assumption that in the past the number of admissions for spontaneous abortion and ectopic pregnancies has been approximately 7% of 'conceptions'.

Table 1.8 given in the last report for England and Wales showed the estimated number of pregnancies by the age of the women from 1972–74 to 1982–84 derived from Table 1.7. Data for 1985–87 have not been included here as the total pregnancies given in Table 1.7 have been estimated. Therefore this report does not include the data given in Table 1.8 in the last England and Wales report.

Figure 1.4a Direct obstetric mortality rate United Kingdom 1976–87

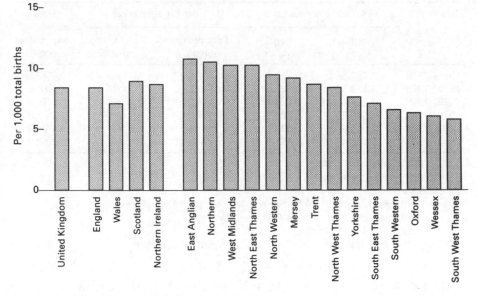

Source: Confidential enquiries into maternal deaths

Figure 1.4b Perinatal mortality rate United Kingdom 1976–87

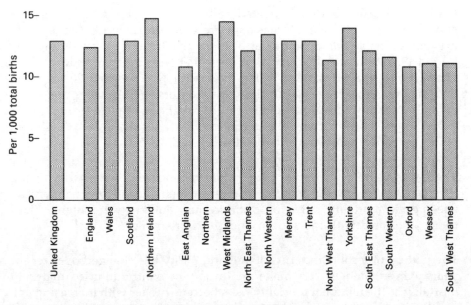

Source: Unpublished data from OPCS, GRO(S) and GRO(NI)

Table 1.7 *Estimated number of pregnancies, residents of England and Wales 1970–87*

(thousands)

Triennium	Estimated conceptions		Hospital admissions		Total estimated pregnancies (000s)
	Maternities	Legal abortions	Spontaneous abortions	Ectopic pregnancies	
1970–1972	2,222.5	290.0	207.6†	11.6	2,732.6
1973–1975	1,852.9	327.9	175.3†	11.7	2,366.8
1976–1978	1,781.3	324.6	158.3†	11.6	2,275.8
1979–1981	1,910.9	380.5	134.3*	12.1	2,437.8
1982–1984	1,905.8	393.1	113.6*	14.4	2,426.9
1985–1987**	2,015.1	451.5	—184.3 combined—		2,650.9

† ICD (8th revision) 640–645
* ICD (9th revision) 634–638
** Estimated
Source: Birth statistics 1837–1983, Series FM1, No 13, Table 12.2.
  Birth statistics 1987, Series FM1, No 16.
  Hospital In-Patient Enquiry
  Note: Conception statistics are based on date of conception.

The demographic characteristics of maternal deaths

Country of birth

Data by country of birth have been presented in earlier reports. Such data, however, are only available for maternities in England and Wales. Also, these latter data are becoming less reliable as an indicator of ethnic origin since birth statistics are unable to identify the increasing number of births to second or later generation immigrant mothers (who are classified as UK born). Therefore it has been decided not to include such data in this report.

Age and parity

Maternal mortality is closely related to both maternal age and parity, as shown by the England and Wales data presented in Table 1.8. Similar data are not available for Scotland and Northern Ireland. Considering the period 1976–87 as a whole, it can be seen that Direct maternal death rates showed a 'J' shaped pattern, being lowest for women aged 20–24 years and then rising with age, particularly for mothers aged 35 years and over. Overall mortality rates for women rise throughout the age group 16–45 years but the contribution of maternal mortality also follows a 'J' shape, being lowest for women aged 20–34 years.

There was a similar pattern of Direct maternal mortality with parity, being 'J' shaped with lowest rates for women in their second pregnancy. The age-specific mortality rates for primiparous mothers were higher than those associated with the second and third pregnancy.

The pattern of fertility in terms of age and parity has changed over recent years. These changes can make an important contribution to maternal mortality as the maternal mortality risks become higher with increasing age and parity. Unfortunately the small number of maternal deaths when

Table 1.8 *Mortality rates of Direct maternal deaths per million maternities by age and parity, England & Wales 1976–87*

Age (years)	Parity						Mortality rates women aged 16–44 years per million population	Percentage of all deaths which are maternal
	1	2	3	4	5+	Total		
under 20	83.0	47.9	—	—	—	77.7	333.3	23.0
20–24	65.3	33.4	39.3	63.1	130.0	52.2	351.1	15.0
25–29	93.4	53.3	77.2	86.7	84.6	75.0	427.6	17.0
30–34	104.4	75.9	92.2	136.4	167.5	99.0	605.1	16.0
35–39	282.8	170.8	181.2	330.4	251.9	229.3	940.2	24.0
40+	638.7	58.3	606.1	619.5	621.4	550.8	1,585.5	34.0
Total	87.9	57.0	91.8	152.7	209.8	86.7	680.9	13.0

analysed by both age and parity means that it is not possible to examine trends over time at this detailed level. Table 1.9, however, shows separately the changes in the age and parity distribution of maternities in England and Wales for every third triennium between 1955–57 and 1982–84 plus those for 1985–87. There has been a decreasing proportion of women having their fourth or more child; 17% of maternities in 1955–57 compared with 10% in 1985–87. More women are delaying childbearing; after a peak in 1964–66 when 67% of women having their first child were aged under 25 years, the age distribution at first birth shifted towards older ages so that by 1985–87 54% of these women were aged under 25 years.

Table 1.9 *Percentage distribution of all maternities by birth order* and age, and by age at first birth, for every previous third triennium, England & Wales only.*

	1955–57	1964–66	1973–75	1982–84	1985–87
Birth order					
1	38	36	40	41	42
2	29	30	36	35	33
3	15	17	14	16	15
4	8	8	5	6	6
5 and over	9	9	4	4	4
Total	100	100	100	100	100
Age (years)					
Under 20	5	10	11	9	9
20–24	29	32	32	30	29
25–29	32	30	37	34	35
30–34	20	17	14	19	20
35–39	10	8	5	6	7
40 and over	3	3	1	1	1
Total	100	100	100	100	100
Age (years) at first birth					
Under 20	12	21	21	18	18
20–24	45	46	39	38	36
25–29	28	23	31	30	31
30–34	11	7	7	11	12
35 and over	4	3	2	3	3
Total	100	100	100	100	100

Source: Unpublished OPCS fertility tables.
* Note: 'Birth order' is defined as the number of live-born children, including the present deliveries, adjusted to convert the number of live births to estimated maternities.

Marital status

Table 1.10 shows the marital status of the women who suffered a Direct or Indirect maternal death in 1985–87, with one quarter of the mothers being unmarried at the time of death. This is consistent with the 23% of live births born outside marriage in 1987 in England and Wales.

Table 1.10 *Maternal deaths in relation to marital status, United Kingdom 1985–87.*

Marital Status	Direct deaths	Indirect deaths	Total	Percentage of series	Percentage maternities*	Rate per million maternities*
Married	105	59	164	73.5	74.0	104.9
Single	21	16	37	16.6	)	)
Widowed	2	—	2	0.9	)	)
Divorced	6	4	10	4.5	) 26.0	) 138.9
Separated	2	3	5	2.2	)	)
Not Stated	3	2	5	2.2		
Total	139	84	223	100	100	

* For England & Wales only.

Review of causes of maternal mortality 1970–87

The two major causes of maternal death in England and Wales since the 1970–72 triennium have been pulmonary embolism and hypertensive disorders of pregnancy. The number and respective percentage of maternal deaths for the relevant triennia between 1970 and 1987 for England and Wales are shown in Table 1.11. It will be noted that, apart from 1982–84 when the numbers and percentages for each condition were identical, hypertensive disorders were the major cause of death in three of the five triennia for England and Wales. The fluctuation in position is even more apparent when the UK triennium for 1985–87 is considered since thromboembolism was the major cause of maternal death (Table 1.12). It is of interest that for England and Wales ectopic pregnancy and haemorrhage (antepartum and postpartum) were the third and fourth major causes of Direct maternal death; neither condition was in the top four in the 1982–84 triennium (Table 1.11). Indeed haemorrhage has not appeared in the top four main causes of maternal death since 1976–78. Although the number of deaths from amniotic fluid embolism has fallen it was the fifth major cause of Direct death. The dramatic reduction in deaths directly due to anaesthesia is demonstrated by the fact that these fell below abortion, sepsis and ruptured uterus. These represented the sixth equal major cause of Direct maternal death. The significance of 'Other Direct causes of death' hides the fact that there were as many deaths from liver disorders in pregnancy as there were from each of abortion, sepsis and ruptured uterus in this triennium for England and Wales.

The new groupings of Direct deaths for the UK make a strict comparison difficult but they are given in Table 1.12. It will be noted that anaesthesia, genital tract trauma and sepsis (excluding abortion) are each the sixth commonest cause of Direct maternal mortality after thromboembolism, hypertensive disorders, early pregnancy deaths, antepartum and postpartum haemorrhage and amniotic fluid embolism.

12

Table 1.11 *Cause of Direct maternal deaths/numbers and percentages, England and Wales 1970–87, compared with United Kingdom, 1985–87.*

Triennium		Cause of Direct maternal death										All deaths
		Pulmonary embolism	Hypertensive disorders of pregnancy	Anaesthesia	Amniotic fluid embolism	Abortion	Ectopic pregnancy	Haemorrhage	Sepsis, excluding abortion	Ruptured uterus	Other direct causes	
England & Wales	1970–72 No.	51	43	37	14	73	34	30	30	11	20	343
	%	14.9	12.5	10.8	4.1	21.3	9.9	8.7	8.7	3.2	5.8	100
	1973–75 No.	33	34	27	14	27	19	21	19	11	22	227
	%	14.5	15.0	11.9	6.2	11.9	8.4	9.3	8.4	4.8	9.7	100
	1976–78 No.	43	29	27	11	14	21	24	15	14	19	217
	%	19.8	13.4	12.4	5.1	6.5	9.7	11.1	6.9	6.5	8.8	100
	1979–81‡ No.	23	36	22	18	14	20	14	8	4	19	178
	%	12.9	20.2	12.4	10.1	7.9	11.2	7.9	4.5	2.2	10.7	100
	1982–84 No.	25	25	18	14	11	10	9	2	3	21	138
	%	18.1	18.1	13.0	10.1	8.0	7.2	6.5	1.4	2.2	15.2	100
	1985–87 No.	24*	25	5	9	6	11	10	6	5**	20***	121
	%	19.8	20.7	4.1	7.4	5.0	9.1	8.3	5.0	4.1	16.5	100
United Kingdom	1985–87 No.	29* ①	27 ②	6	9	6	16	10	6	6**	24†	139
	%	20.9	19.4	4.3	6.5	4.3	11.5	7.2	4.3	4.3	17.3	100

*   excluding deaths following abortion
**   including other genital tract trauma
***   includes 2 thrombosis deaths
‡   includes two other Direct deaths omitted in the 1976–78 report.
†   includes 3 deaths from thrombosis and 1 Direct cardiac death.

Table 1.12 *Cause of Direct maternal deaths/numbers and percentages, United Kingdom 1985–87.*

	Thrombosis and thrombo-embolism	Hypertensive disorders of pregnancy	Anaesthesia	Amniotic fluid embolism	Early pregnancy deaths (including abortion)	Antepartum and postpartum haemorrhage	Genital tract sepsis (excluding abortion)	Genital tract trauma	Other Direct deaths	All deaths
No.	32*	27	6	9	22	10	6	6	21**	139
%	23.0	19.4	4.3	6.5	15.8	7.2	4.3	4.3	15.1	100

* Excluding 1 death following abortion, but including 3 deaths from thrombosis
** Including 1 Direct cardiac death.

Table 1.13 *Direct deaths by cause, rates per million estimated pregnancies, England and Wales 1970–87†.*

Triennium	Cause of Direct maternal death										
	Pulmonary embolism	Hypertensive diseases of pregnancy	Anaesthesia	Amniotic fluid embolism	Abortion	Ectopic pregnancy	Haemorrhage	Sepsis, excluding abortion	Ruptured uterus	Other direct causes	All deaths
1970–72	17.6	14.9	12.8	4.8	25.3	11.5	10.4	10.4	3.8	6.9	118.7
1973–75	12.8	13.2	10.5	5.4	10.5	7.4	8.1	7.4	4.3	8.5	88.0
1976–78	18.5	12.5	11.6	4.7	6.0	9.0	10.3	6.5	6.0	8.2	93.4
1979–81*	9.0	14.2	8.7	7.1	5.5	7.9	5.5	3.1	1.6	7.5	70.0*
1982–84	10.0	10.0	7.2	5.6	4.4	4.0	3.6	1.0	1.2	8.4	55.0
1985–87	9.1	9.4	1.9	3.4	2.3	4.1	3.8	2.3	1.9	7.5	45.6

* Includes two other Direct deaths omitted in the 1976–78 Report.

† Rates for the United Kingdom were not available as there was no information on pregnancies for Scotland and Northern Ireland.

15

Table 1.13 indicates the death rate for Direct maternal deaths per million pregnancies between 1970 and 1987 for England and Wales. It will be noted when considering all deaths that the rate for all Direct deaths was 93.4 in 1976–78 and it was 45.6 in 1985–87. The fall in deaths between the triennium 1985–87 compared with 1982–84 is slight, but is of approximately similar order to that noted between each triennium, the fall being between 20–25% in each of the triennia. When one compares the death rate for each condition it will be noted that the most dramatic falls have been in abortion deaths and anaesthetic deaths. Whilst the abortion deaths can be related to the introduction of the 1967 Abortion Act, the fall in anaesthetic deaths is undoubtedly due to the improved services provided by the obstetric anaesthetists. Their highly critical appraisal of the care of the obstetric patients who required anaesthesia in this report nevertheless indicates the possibilities for further improvement.

It is apparent from our detailed analysis of maternal deaths that in many instances they reflect deficiencies in the maternity services available. Failure of communication of potential problems to more senior and experienced midwives, doctors, obstetricians or anaesthetists is often noted. A reappraisal of the total staff, midwifery and medical, available to provide adequate cover on a 24-hour basis is required by all units and there should be a regular review of the service available. The avoidance of split sites in any future planning is essential, as is a greater involvement of consultants during pregnancy and labour.

Each of the causes of maternal death are considered separately in the following chapters.

References

1 Hogberg U. Maternal mortality — a world wide problem. *Int J Gynaecol Obstet* 1985; 23: 463–470.
2 Editorial. Maternal Health in Subsaharan Africa. *Lancet* 1987; i: 255–257.

CHAPTER 2

Hypertensive disorders of pregnancy

Summary

The number of deaths due to hypertensive disorders in the United Kingdom (UK) during the triennium 1985–87 was 27. This can be compared with 25 for England and Wales only during the triennium 1982–84, and shows that hypertensive disorders of pregnancy remain a major cause of death despite recent advances in the control of hypertension and convulsive disease. Delegation of the initial care in hospital of these cases to junior medical staff, and lack of communication between medical, midwifery and administrative staff at all levels, are important contributary and preventable causes of this type of maternal mortality. It is only too apparent that the recommendations set out in the last two reports for England and Wales, on the establishment and use of specialised Regional Teams to assist in the management of these often difficult cases, have not been generally implemented. This should be done without further delay.

The title of this chapter has been altered, replacing 'diseases' by 'disorders' to conform with the clinical classification devised by the International Society for the Study of Hypertension in Pregnancy, but the well established terms 'pre-eclampsia' and 'eclampsia' have been retained. These two related disorders were responsible for all 27 deaths. In 26 the blood pressure was normal in early pregnancy and in only one was essential hypertension present before the onset of pregnancy.

The number of women who died from hypertensive disorders of pregnancy and the death rate per million maternities for the years 1970–87 inclusive in England and Wales are compared with those for the United Kingdom in 1985–87 in Table 2.1.

Table 2.1 *Number of women who died from hypertensive disorders of pregnancy and the death rate per million maternities, England and Wales 1970–87, compared with United Kingdom 1985–87.*

	Triennium	Total		Pre-eclampsia		Eclampsia	
		Number	Rate	Number	Rate	Number	Rate
England	1970–72	43	18.7	14	6.1	29	12.6
& Wales	1973–75	34	17.7	15	7.8	19	9.9
	1976–78	29	16.6	16	9.1	13	7.4
	1979–81	36	18.7	16	8.3	20	10.4
	1982–84	25	13.3	11	5.8	14	7.4
	1985–87	25	12.6	13	6.5	12	6.0
United Kingdom	1985–87	27	12.1	15	6.7	12	5.4

Table 2.2 Number of maternal deaths and the death rates per million maternities from hypertensive disorders by age, England and Wales 1970–87, compared with United Kingdom 1985–87.

Age (years)	1970–84 England and Wales			1985–87 England and Wales			1985–87 United Kingdom		
	Maternities total (000s)	No. of deaths	Rate per million	Maternities total (000s)	No. of deaths	Rate per million	Maternities total (000s)	No. of deaths	Rate per million
Under 25	4,113.5	62	15.1	749.2	10	13.3	837.8	10	11.9
25–29	3,374.9	53	15.7	691.0	5	7.2	777.7	5	6.4
30–34	1,636.9	28	17.1	389.9	6	15.4	437.6	7	16.0
35–39	528.1	19	36.0	135.1	3	22.2	152.1	3	19.7
40+	122.8	5	40.7	23.6	1	42.4	26.6	2	75.1
All ages	9,776.1	167	17.1	1,987.9	25	12.6	2,231.8	27	12.1

It will be noted that the number of deaths and death rates from pre-eclampsia in England and Wales remained similar between 1970–72 and 1985–87 whereas the numbers of deaths and death rates from eclampsia have in general fallen.

A comparison of the age of women who died of hypertensive disorders of pregnancy in 1970–87 in England and Wales with those who died in 1985–87 in the United Kingdom is given in Table 2.2.

The influence of age, particularly 35 years and over, is apparent.

Pre-eclampsia and eclampsia (1985–87)

Severe pre-eclampsia was present in 15 cases and eclampsia in 12. In seven other women pre-eclampsia was a factor but the deaths were considered to be directly due to other conditions and counted in Chapters on Haemorrhage, Thrombosis and thromboembolism, Cardiac disease, Anaesthesia and there were two Indirect deaths.

In 1985–87 only one young parous woman died undelivered.

> Her weight had increased by 19kg and her blood pressure had risen from 110/70 to 135/90 mm Hg by the 28th week of pregnancy. When seen by her general practitioner a week later her blood pressure was 140/90 mm Hg and she had heavy (+ +) proteinuria. A hospital appointment was made for the next day, but early that morning she developed signs of placental abruption and was immediately admitted to hospital. This diagnosis was confirmed by the senior house officer (SHO) on duty. The fetal heart was still audible and an IV infusion of hydralazine and diazepam was commenced. Blood was sent for cross-matching and clotting studies. Three hours later artificial rupture of the membranes revealed bloodstained amniotic fluid. She was then seen by the consultant obstetrician for the first time when the fetal heart was inaudible and clotting studies indicated disseminated intravascular coagulation (DIC). Caesarean section was considered at this stage and a senior house officer anaesthetist set up a central venous line with difficulty which 'appeared to be working'. After discussion with the consultant anaesthetist it was decided to defer Caesarean section until the arrival of blood and platelets from a distant blood transfusion unit. The DIC worsened rapidly and 2½ hours after she was first seen by the consultant anaesthetist she collapsed with signs of pulmonary oedema. A consultant physician as well as the obstetrician and anaesthetist attempted to resuscitate her. Despite intubation, manual ventilation and, eventually, external cardiac massage she died undelivered 50 minutes later. Whilst the autopsy confirmed the diagnosis of massive placental abruption and DIC with large confluent pulmonary haemorrhages, no histology was recorded.

The duration of pregnancy at delivery is shown in Table 2.3.

Twenty-six women died after delivery.

19

Table 2.3 *Duration of pregnancy at delivery*

Duration of pregnancy (weeks)	Pre-eclampsia	Eclampsia	Total
Up to 28	2	1	3
29–32	2	4	6
33–37	6	4	10
38–40	4	3	7

Ten of the 27 deaths (37%), including the woman who died undelivered, occurred before the thirty-third week; five women had severe pre-eclampsia and five had eclampsia.

There were nine spontaneous cephalic deliveries and one breech delivery. One infant was delivered with forceps and the remaining 15 by Caesarean section.

Perinatal mortality

There was one intrauterine death in the woman who died undelivered at 29 weeks; five stillbirths, all after 28 weeks; and four neonatal deaths, three before and one after 28 weeks gestation. This perinatal mortality, 10 out of 27 or a rate of 370 per 1,000, may be compared with a rate of 263 per 1,000 during 1982–84 and 333 per 1,000 during 1979–81 in England and Wales. The fetal prognosis in hypertensive disorders when maternal death occurs has obviously not improved during the past nine years.

Eclamptic fits

Six women had convulsions before treatment of pre-eclampsia was begun. Of the other six who had their first convulsion in hospital, one woman was antenatal, one was in labour and four were postpartum. The importance of careful surveillance of pre-eclamptic patients in the early puerperium cannot be overstressed. Fits were not always controlled by the initial treatment and multiple convulsions (four or more) occurred in five women prior to the onset of labour. (Table 2.4)

Table 2.4 *Number and timing of eclamptic fits*

Number of fits	Antepartum	Postpartum	Total
1	1	3	4
2	1	1	2
3	0	1	1
4	5	0	5

It is of note that eight of the 12 women had two or more fits. It is possible that prompt and effective treatment of the first fit might have been life saving.

Pathology

Autopsies were performed in 25 of the 27 deaths but only 18 were regarded as adequate. In 12 histological information was not available or was unsatisfactory. Of the two cases where autopsy was not performed, one had clinical evidence of cerebral haemorrhage complicating severe pre-eclampsia ten hours after delivery and the other had severe pre-eclampsia with DIC and haemorrhagic pancreatitis confirmed at laparotomy.

Immediate cause of death

Of the 25 autopsies performed 13 were on women with pre-eclampsia and 12 with eclampsia. The immediate causes of death in all 27 cases are show in Table 2.5. There was associated DIC in 12 women.

Table 2.5 *Immediate cause of death*

Cause of death	Totals	Pre-eclampsia	Eclampsia
Pulmonary complication	12	4	8
Intracerebral haemorrhage	11	7	4
Acute pancreatitis	1	1	—
Ruptured aortic aneurysm	1	1	—
Renal failure	1	1	—
Hepatorenal failure	1	1	—
	27	15	12

In the triennium 1982–84 for England and Wales the immediate cause of death was cerebral complications in 21 women, pulmonary oedema, due to IV fluid overload, in three, and hepatic necrosis in one (Table 2.6). In 1985–87 there has thus been a striking increase in the occurrence of death due to pulmonary complications especially adult respiratory distress syndrome (ARDS) which is noted for the first time in the Confidential Enquiries and occurred nine times.

The other pulmonary cases in 1979–87 (Table 2.6) include four cases of pulmonary oedema, one due to IV fluid overload, two of bronchopneumonia and one case each of pulmonary haemorrhage and hydrothorax.

Substandard care

Care was considered to be substandard in 23 of the 27 cases (81%). The cause of this was attributed to the woman herself in four; to the general practitioner in three; to the general practitioner and the hospital staff jointly in two; and to the hospital obstetric team in 14.

Patient responsibility

The main factors here were failure to attend hospital when requested and refusal to accept medical advice, and two examples are given.

Table 2.6 *Causes of death 1979–87*

Cause of death	England and Wales 1979–81	England and Wales 1982–84	UK 1985–87
Cerebral	17	21	11
Haemorrhage	10	14	11
Necrosis	2	3	0
Oedema	5	4	0
Pulmonary	2	3	12
Adult respiratory distress			
syndrome	0	0	9
Oedema	0	3	1
Hydrothorax	1	0	0
Haemorrhage	0	0	1
Bronchopneumonia	1	0	1
Hepatic			
Necrosis	8	0	1
Other	9	1	3
Total	36	25	27

A young normotensive parous woman developed moderate (+) proteinuria at 36 weeks. She defaulted from the antenatal clinic the following week and when seen a week later showed evidence of severe pre-eclampsia with marked oedema, raised blood pressure and heavy (+ +) proteinuria. She was admitted that evening and after commencing anti-hypertensive treatment labour was induced next afternoon. Three hours later recurrent fits began and despite delivery by Caesarean section and appropriate anti-hypertensive and anticonvulsive therapy in the intensive care unit (ICU) she developed pulmonary oedema, irreversible cardiac arrest and died 16 hours after delivery.

A parous woman who developed marked hypertension (180/110 mm Hg) at 30 weeks refused to come into hospital. Anti-hypertensive therapy was prescribed but not taken. At 32 weeks she agreed to come in but, having been allowed home for a weekend, failed to return. She was admitted when she re-attended at 37 weeks with fulminating pre-eclampsia. Despite appropriate anti-hypertensive treatment and delivery by Caesarean section, she failed to improve and died of cerebral haemorrhage.

General practitioner responsibility

Antenatal care by the general practitioner was adjudged substandard on three occasions and the following case is one example.

A parous woman was found to have hypertension, oedema and heavy (+ + +) proteinuria at 33 weeks. She was advised by her general practitioner to rest at home. Two days later she developed status eclampticus, inhaled vomit and died 10 days later in the ICU with ARDS.

General practitioner and hospital staff responsibility

This was considered a major factor in two cases.

A parous woman was noted by her general practitioner to have a trace of proteinuria, and a blood pressure of 130/84 mm Hg. No action was taken and several days later she had an eclamptic fit. Her general practitioner did not visit her but arranged for her admission to a hospital half a mile away from the obstetric unit. She was taken unsedated to a Medical Unit and had two fits en route. A junior obstetric staff member made a diagnosis of a neurological condition without testing her urine and sent her to the medical intensive therapy unit. She was over-sedated with drugs rarely used in obstetric practice and grossly over-loaded with IV fluids. She was delivered spontaneously of a stillborn baby girl and died 48 hours after admission from cardiovascular failure due to eclampsia, complicated by aspiration of vomit.

In the case of the woman who died undelivered, the significance of excessive weight gain associated with rising blood pressure was not appreciated. When the sinister development of heavy proteinuria occurred this was not regarded as requiring immediate admission to hospital. After admission with placental abruption the care of this dangerously ill woman was left in the hands of the duty obstetric and anaesthetic SHOs for several hours before the consultant obstetrician could be contacted. After the consultant obstetrician and anaesthetists were involved Caesarean section, although decided upon, was deferred until too late because blood and platelets had to be obtained from a blood transfusion unit over 20 miles away.

Consultant unit responsibility

The largest group, 14 out of the 23 cases where care was substandard, was the responsibility of the consultant obstetric unit. In these cases there were two main defects involved:–

a. Inappropriate delegation of clinical responsibility.

b. Undue delay in making or implementing critical clinical decisions.

a. *Inappropriate delegation*

Junior obstetric staff as mentioned in these examples were either allowed to take important decisions without consultation or to undertake major surgery in high risk patients.

A parous woman had had a previous Caesarean section. She was admitted at 34 weeks with severe pre-eclampsia. Her hypertension was controlled with IV Hydralazine. She was delivered by emergency Caesarean section by an SHO assisted by the senior registrar. The previous transverse suprapubic incision had been reopened and severe haemorrhage from the right inferior epigastric artery subsequently required repeat laparotomy for haemostasis after an estimated blood loss of two litres.

Resuscitation was undertaken in the ICU but pulmonary oedema occurred requiring prolonged assisted ventilation and tracheotomy under anaesthesia. Uterine sepsis was suspected and subtotal hysterectomy performed by the senior registrar. No uterine sepsis was found and postoperatively it became increasingly difficult to ventilate her. She died two weeks after the Caesarean section. The autopsy indicated that the immediate cause of death was bronchopneumonia secondary to prolonged ventilation and repeated general anaesthesia.

In two other cases obstetric SHOs prescribed inadequate treatment for high risk patients over the telephone without examining them. Their condition deteriorated rapidly and despite subsequent energetic therapy both died a few hours later, one with eclampsia and DIC, the other with severe pre-eclampsia and massive intracerebral haemorrhage.

b. Undue delay

In some cases there was a failure to appreciate the gravity of the maternal condition and delivery was deferred because of the immaturity of the fetus.

A highly parous woman developed severe pre-eclampsia at 23 weeks gestation. Despite treatment in hospital her condition continued to deteriorate. Nevertheless delivery by hysterotomy was delayed for several days. Postoperatively she failed to respond to treatment and died of renal failure complicating severe pre-eclampsia, a week later.

Implementation of decisions already taken was sometimes delayed because of administrative and clinical deficiencies. The disastrous results of such procrastination are very apparent in such cases as the last case described above, and the patient who died undelivered.

Anaesthetic involvement

Anaesthesia or sedation was considered to have contributed to three deaths. Two died secondary to complications within the first two hours after emergency Caesarean section, and the third received excessive sedation when labour was induced at only 26 weeks gestation. These cases are detailed in Chapter 9.

Anaesthetic staff should be involved early in the management of women with severe pre-eclampsia, even if operative delivery is not planned, to assist with analgesia, sedation, anti-hypertensive therapy and monitoring. Epidural anaesthesia is commonly used to decrease blood pressure in labouring patients with pre-eclampsia. It probably acts by diminishing pain and anxiety and by reducing vasomotor tone. However epidural anaesthesia takes some time to be established and fails to control blood pressure in women with severe disease. In such cases the additional use of anti-hypertensive drugs is required. In women with severe pre-eclampsia and a reduced circulatory volume epidural anaesthesia may cause marked arterial hypotension. Careful fluid replacement, if necessary under central venous pressure monitoring, is advisable.

The choice of anaesthetic technique for operative delivery in women with severe pre-eclampsia is influenced by the maternal and fetal condition and the urgency of delivery. If general anaesthesia is indicated consideration should always be given to the possibility of a hypertensive response to tracheal intubation.

In the postoperative period when the effects of general or epidural anaesthesia subside sympathetic tone returns. If significant volumes of fluid have been given during anaesthesia, the circulation may become overloaded. Careful monitoring of arterial and central venous pressure for at least 12 hours after operation, particularly if anti-hypertensive therapy is continued, is essential. The haemodynamic status of such patients before, during and after delivery is complex and anaesthetists and obstetricians in training should receive formal instruction in this difficult aspect of care.

A large number of the cases in this chapter were managed in an ICU with prolonged periods of artificial ventilation. Nine women died of ARDS. Whilst ventilation was indicated initially in most of these cases because of ventilatory failure due to eclampsia, heavy sedation, or unrecognised aspiration of gastric contents it was generally continued because of worsening gas exchange in the lungs due to alveolar membrane dysfunction and pulmonary oedema. It is possible that careful monitoring of arterial pressure and right and left filling pressures with restriction of fluid intake might reduce the incidence of ARDS in these patients.

Assistance from cardiac, renal, haematological and other physicians as well as specialised surgeons can be of great assistance in managing difficult obstetric problems. However for this to be so requires that the specialists involved should have wide experience in treating complications of pregnancy, otherwise advice may be given that is inappropriate. This was judged to have occurred in four cases in this series of maternal deaths:—

1. Anti-hypertensive therapy was reduced too precipitately and too soon in the puerperium in a woman with severe pre-eclampsia; and eclampsia supervened.

2. Liver complications were not at first recognised as pre-eclamptic in origin and appropriate treatment was not instituted.

3. Unorthodox ineffective anticonvulsants were used by non-obstetric staff in an ICU.

4. A medical registrar prescribed anticoagulants in a severely pre-eclamptic patient with chest pain in the puerperium and precipitated fatal cerebral haemorrhage.

Discussion

In the last report for England and Wales 1982–84 a welcome reduction was noted in the number of maternal deaths due to hypertensive disorders to 25, compared with 36 in 1979–81. It is disappointing that during 1985–87 there was no fall in mortality, and that the percentage of cases where care was judged to be substandard has risen from 72 to 81.

This lack of progress can still be ascribed to failure at all levels of care involving the pregnant women themselves as well as those responsible for their obstetric care. Pregnant women and their relatives must be advised of the risk of pre-eclampsia to them and their babies.

The natural desire of a woman, feeling relatively normal, to return home to her family; or her failure to attend the antenatal clinic regularly, can have dire consequences for her. Whilst it is possible that at least in the earlier stages of pre-eclampsia home care might be more widely used in suitable cases, this requires careful organisation and supervision with regular examination of the patient to detect any signs or symptoms of deterioration, and if necessary to arrange immediate admission to hospital. General practitioners practising antenatal care should always be alert to the risks of even apparently mild pre-eclampsia.

The consultant in charge of the hospital obstetric team should emphasise to all his/her staff the importance of hypertensive disorders at all stages of pregnancy, ante-, intra- and postpartum.

This can best be accomplished by insisting that in every case and at all hours, women with moderate or severe pre-eclampsia, whether seen initially or during observation in hospital, be examined, as a matter of urgency, by a consultant obstetrician whose duty it is to determine the immediate and subsequent management in detail.

Junior members of the obstetric team should not be permitted or expected to make executive decisions in such cases. They should be made acutely aware of the potentially disastrous nature of these disorders and recognise that their duty is to inform their seniors of such cases immediately they are encountered.

Once again it must be reiterated, as in previous reports, that because fulminating pre-eclampsia and eclampsia are now rarely seen in the UK, it is essential if maternal mortality from these disorders is to be reduced further, that local specialised teams should be set up in all Regions to deal with such patients either in an advisory capacity or, where necessary, directly in fully equipped and staffed high dependency areas in the obstetric unit preferably near the labour ward.

These teams should include, along with experienced obstetricians and obstetric anaesthetists, physicians expert in hypertensive and renal disorders, who would take a special interest, and acquire wide experience, in the management of these difficult obstetrical cases.

The organisation of these specialist teams should be the responsibility of a senior obstetric consultant in each Region. He should supervise the staffing of the team and, after consultation with all interested parties, determine the standing orders relating to such matters as transport, under direct medical supervision, of patients to hospital in an emergency and the regimens and drugs used to control blood pressure and convulsions before and after admission to hospital. In this way it may be possible to reduce if not abolish the occurrence of eclamptic fits in women under medical supervision such as was seen in half of the eclamptics in this triennium. Early and continuing expert supervision should also go a long way towards eliminating the defects and delays that have contributed to the present maternal mortality.

Drugs

Diazepam and chlormethiazole were the drugs commonly used for the control of convulsions, as was hydralazine for hypertension, in this series. It should be recognised that diazepam alone is not a good anticonvulsant and it should be used intravenously to control a fit but not relied on to prevent recurrent eclamptic convulsions. Magnesium sulphate still fails to gain popularity in the United Kingdom. Perhaps its use should be scientifically re-evaluated. Intravenous phenytoin may have a place in the prophylaxis of eclamptic convulsions in susceptible women and should also continue to be assessed.

There has been a striking increase in this triennium in the number of deaths from pulmonary complication which were the immediate cause of death in 12 out of the 27 deaths. This is the first time that the occurrence of ARDS in patients dying from a hypertensive disorder has been noted in these reports. There were nine deaths from this cause and this occurred 4–21 (average 13) days after delivery. It is possible that patients who might previously have died at an earlier stage from severe cerebral complications are now, as a result of modern techniques of resuscitation, living long enough to develop changes in the lungs, perhaps aggravated by fluid imbalance, leading to interference with exchange of blood gases and eventually death from hypoxia and multi-organ failure. An in-depth, possible multi-centre study of this would seem to be indicated.

The outcome for the baby has also not improved in the past nine years. In this triennium there were six stillbirths and four neonatal deaths. Earlier Caesarean section might have salvaged some of these and the importance of early and full involvement of perinatal expertise is obvious in dealing with small hypoxic babies such as these.

CHAPTER 3

Antepartum and postpartum haemorrhage

Summary

This chapter replaces that headed 'Haemorrhage' in previous reports. Only deaths due to haemorrhage from the genital tract are included here; deaths due to haemorrhage from other sites are considered in the relevant chapters.

Of the 10 deaths directly due to antepartum and postpartum haemorrhage, four were caused by placental abruption and six by postpartum haemorrhage. There were no Direct deaths due to placenta praevia and no Late deaths. Care was substandard in seven of the 10 deaths. In addition to these 10 Direct deaths bleeding was implicated in 12 other deaths which are dealt with in their relevant chapters (5, 8 and 12).

Haemorrhage

In 1985–87 there were 10 Direct deaths from haemorrhage with a mortality rate of 4.5 per million maternities. There were no Late deaths. Of these 10 Direct deaths four were caused by placental abruption (ICD 641) and six by postpartum haemorrhage (ICD 666). Care was considered substandard in seven compared with six of the nine in 1982–4 and 12 out of 14 in 1979–81 in England and Wales.

Table 3.1 shows the number of Direct deaths from haemorrhage by cause and the death rate per million maternities in the six triennia from 1970–72 in England and Wales and the triennium from 1985–87 in the United Kingdom (UK). In addition to the 10 Direct deaths discussed in this chapter there were 12 from other causes in which bleeding played a significant part. These are considered in their relevant chapters. Antepartum haemorrhage from placenta praevia treated by Caesarean section was followed by death in two cases — one directly attributable to pulmonary embolism, (Chapter 4), the other due to cardiac disease (Chapter 11). Antepartum haemorrhage with coagulation failure due to placental abruption occurred in one of the deaths directly attributable to a hypertensive disorder (Chapter 2). Two more of the latter deaths were complicated by postpartum haemorrhage following Caesarean section (Chapter 13). Postpartum haemorrhage also occurred in a patient who died of amniotic fluid embolism (Chapter 5) and all six deaths directly attributable to genital tract trauma (Chapter 8).

The death rate by age per million maternities given in Table 3.2 indicates an increased risk with age but particularly for those aged 35 years and over. The overall rate is about 5 per million maternities judged by the last three triennial reports for England and Wales.

Table 3.1 *Number of deaths from haemorrhage and rates per million maternities, England and Wales 1970–87 compared with United Kingdom 1985–87.*

	Triennium	Placental abruption	Placenta praevia	Postpartum haemorrhage	Total	Rate per million maternities
England	1970–72	6	6	18	30	13.1
& Wales	1973–75	6	2	13	21	10.9
	1976–78	6	2	16	24	13.7
	1979–81	2	3	9	14	7.3
	1982–84	2	2	3	7	3.5
	1985–87	4	0	6	10	5.0
United Kingdom	1985–87	4	0	6	10	4.5

Four maternal deaths were caused directly by placental abruption, which was preceded by pre-eclampsia in one instance. One patient died undelivered; two had spontaneous deliveries of dead fetuses; the fourth was delivered by Caesarean section and the baby survived. Severe coagulopathy was diagnosed clinically in three of these patients and confirmed at autopsy in two.

Care was considered to be substandard in three cases. The first developed renal failure and was overloaded with IV fluids. The second was inadequately resuscitated because the degree of exsanguination was not appreciated and experienced help was sought too late.

A woman with intrauterine fetal death was admitted in labour and was seen by the resident obstetric staff. Blood loss after a spontaneous delivery was 750ml. The consultant was informed at this stage but did not see the patient until two hours later. Meanwhile bleeding continued and hypovolaemic shock developed. However, blood was not available for another 75 minutes, when her haemoglobin concentration was 5.0g/dl, and only 1 litre was administered over a period of one hour, at which time cardiac arrest occurred. She was treated by the cardiac arrest team but despite intensive resuscitative measures cardiac arrest occurred a second time and she died within 12 hours of delivery.

Autopsy revealed extensive haemorrhage into the body cavities but no microscopic evidence of disseminated intravascular coagulation (DIC) despite the clinical history of a clotting defect.

The third death was mainly attributable to the patient's religious scruples which prevented adequate resuscitation.

A parous woman was admitted following placental abruption at 36 weeks gestation. After a spontaneous labour she had a postpartum haemorrhage of one litre. In spite of defective coagulation and severe anaemia she refused blood or blood products on religious grounds. Exploration of the uterus showed no retained products or rupture and packing failed to control the bleeding. Abdominal hysterectomy was therefore performed about three hours after delivery and at the end of the procedure the haemoglobin concentration was 3.4g/dl. She was transferred by ambulance to an adjacent intensive care unit, where she

Table 3.2 The number of deaths from haemorrhage, and death rates per million maternities by age from haemorrhage, England and Wales 1970–84, compared with United Kingdom 1985–87.

Age (years)	1970–84 England and Wales			1985–87 England and Wales			1985–87 United Kingdom		
	Maternities total (000s)	No. of deaths	Rate per million	Maternities total (000s)	No. of deaths	Rate per million	Maternities total (000s)	No. of deaths	Rate per million
Under 25	4,113.5	24	5.8	749.2	4	5.3	837.8	4	4.8
25–29	3,374.9	23	6.8	691.0	—	—	777.7	—	—
30–34	1,636.9	24	14.7	388.9	2	5.1	437.6	2	4.6
35–39	528.1	15	28.4	135.1	3	22.2	152.1	3	19.7
40 +	122.8	12	97.7	23.6	1	42.4	26.6	1	37.5
All ages	9,776.1	98	10.0	1,987.9	10	5	2,231.8	10	4.5

died on the third day of the puerperium. Autopsy showed the features of DIC and adult respiratory distress syndrome (ARDS).

The fourth death directly attributable to haemorrhage from placental abruption is unusual. The woman was apparently leaning over a bath tub washing clothes when she sustained a massive retroplacental haemorrhage and fell into the bath head first and drowned. This singular combination of events would seem to have been unavoidable.

Postpartum haemorrhage

Six deaths were directly caused by postpartum haemorrhage. Four of these were associated with Caesarean section, one with retained products, and one with Factor VIII deficiency.

Of the four associated with Caesarean section care was regarded as sub-standard in three.

A woman who had had a previous Caesarean section, following a reversal of sterilisation operation was admitted with spontaneous rupture of the membranes at 33 weeks. Several days later fetal distress occurred and a Caesarean section was performed by the locum registrar. The placental site was not recorded but there was more than average blood loss, partly from vascularised adhesions. After abdominal closure there was a sudden 'flood of blood' from the vagina not controlled by oxytocics or bimanual compression. The consultant arrived 10 minutes later, when the abdomen had already been reopened. Profuse bleeding was occurring from multiple points inside and outside the uterus and a diagnosis of coagulation failure was made. Resuscitation with blood, frozen plasma, human plasma protein fraction and platelets was begun and hyster-ectomy was performed. This having failed to control the bleeding the internal iliac arteries were ligated and the pelvis was packed. The patient was then transferred to an adjacent intensive care unit (ICU) where resuscitation continued. Nevertheless bleeding persisted and the abdomen was again opened and contained over two litres of blood and clot. Partial haemostasis was achieved with thrombin packs but her condition continued to deteriorate and she died the day after delivery.

At autopsy there were over five litres of fluid blood and clot in the peritoneal cavity and generalised evidence of coagulation defect. It would appear that in this difficult case haemostasis at Caesarean section was inadequate and the initial blood loss was seriously underestimated. No cross-matched blood was immediately available although the operation had been planned, and the blood bank was situated at a distance. The resuscitative measures were inadequate and the coagulopathy was never properly controlled, so that the appropriate surgical efforts to achieve haemostasis failed. In retrospect it is possible that, had the consultant performed the Caesarean section as planned, the fatal outcome would have been prevented.

A parous woman with mild pre-eclampsia at term was delivered by

Caesarean section for fetal distress. There was severe bleeding during and after the operation and blood replacement was delayed and inadequate. Her condition deteriorated rapidly and she died in hypovolaemic shock four and a half hours after delivery. The consultant was not informed until after her death. At autopsy there was 2.5 litres of blood in the uterus and vagina.

In this case the lack of communication with senior staff, the failure to appreciate the degree of haemorrhage, to control it and to replace the blood loss adequately and the poor postoperative supervision must be regarded as substandard care.

A woman of short stature was delivered by Caesarean section by a senior house officer (SHO) acting as registrar after unsuccessful attempts at forceps delivery. Subsequently she became shocked and at laparotomy was found to have a large left broad ligament haematoma. Hysterectomy was required to control bleeding and she was transferred to an adjacent hospital for intensive care. Three weeks later she died of adult respiratory distress syndrome (ARDS).

A parous woman with congenital dislocation of the hips was delivered by Caesarean section with considerable difficulty because of her stiff hips and adhesions from previous surgery. On the second postoperative day she developed a large left broad ligament haematoma which was treated conservatively by blood transfusion. However three days later severe intraperitoneal and extraperitoneal bleeding recurred and was confirmed by laparotomy. Despite the assistance of a vascular surgeon the bleeding could not be arrested and the patient died on the operating table. Autopsy failed to identify any source of haemorrhage.

Two other deaths from postpartum haemorrhage followed normal delivery.

A woman of high parity was delivered at term after a short labour lasting five and a half hours. *Syntometrine* 1 ml was given after the birth of the anterior shoulder. The placenta was removed by controlled cord traction and was thought to be complete. She lost 850 ml of blood and required ergometrine 0.5 mg IM repeated IV after seven minutes. There was no further bleeding and she went home after 48 hours. In the second postpartum week she was readmitted with an estimated secondary postpartum haemorrhage of 600 ml.

Her haemoglobin concentration was then 11.9 g/dl and her condition was good, with a BP of 120/90 mm Hg. Curettage produced copious products of conception and a blood loss of 350 ml. Intravenous *syntocinon* was infused but over the next 12 hours she continued to lose blood. She refused blood transfusion on religious grounds and Haemaccel was commenced. She was seen by the consultant obstetrician the day after admission. Blood transfusion was again advised but refused by the patient and her husband. Bleeding persisted and three hours later her pulse rose to 110/min and her blood pressure fell to 80/50 mm Hg. At this stage she consented to surgery including hysterectomy but steadfastly refused blood transfusion. Her haemoglobin concentration was now 4g/dl and uterine exploration produced 600 ml of clot and fresh severe bleeding. Hysterectomy was performed but her condition deteriorated rapidly, her haemoglobin falling to 1.4 g/dl. Irreversible cardiac arrest occurred and she died the second day after hysterectomy.

As with the third death due to placental abruption described above, this patient's death was largely caused by her religious scruples and refusal of blood transfusion. The secondary postpartum haemorrhage however might have been avoided had the retention of part of the placenta been recognised and treated immediately after delivery. It is possible also that earlier hysterectomy and appropriate monitoring and resuscitation might have saved this patient's life.

A parous woman was admitted to hospital with pre-eclampsia at 36 weeks gestation. Routine blood investigation led to the diagnosis of previously unsuspected Factor VIII deficiency. Following a normal delivery she sustained a postpartum haemorrhage which was treated successfully with two units of blood and fresh frozen plasma. Five days later she bled again and when the haemorrhage could not be controlled hysterectomy was performed. However the bleeding persisted and despite energetic resuscitative measures including massive blood transfusion and Factor VIII replacement she died under intensive care two weeks after delivery.

Autopsy showed massive generalised haemorrhages with bilateral pulmonary collapse, congestive cardiac failure and cerebral oedema, the result of a haemorrhagic diathesis caused by the presence of Factor VIII antibody.

This was a difficult case but it is possible that early treatment of the abnormal clotting state with steroids, immunoglobulin or plasmapheresis might have prevented the fatal outcome.

Coagulation failure

Abnormalities of coagulation were diagnosed clinically in three out of the four placental abruptions and confirmed at autopsy in two. Coagulation defects were diagnosed clinically and confirmed at autopsy in four of the six postpartum haemorrhages including one patient with previously undiagnosed Factor VIII deficiency.

Substandard care

Care was judged to be substandard in three out of four placental abruptions and in four out of the six postpartum haemorrhages. Resuscitation was deficient in six women, two of whom for religious reasons refused blood or blood products which might have been life saving. The other deficiencies could be ascribed mainly to inexperience on the part of the doctors originally in charge of the patient, delay in appreciating the severity of the blood loss, delay in calling more senior assistance or delay in the response of consultants to a call for assistance. Obstetric practice was questionable in one instance where several attempts at forceps delivery were made prior to Caesarean section in a patient of small stature.

Pathology

Autopsy reports were available in nine of the 10 deaths due to haemorrhage. One of the nine reports was considered inadequate. Other defects noted in various reports included failure to provide an adequate histology report, to comment on a hysterectomy specimen, to record relevant organ weights and to conclude the report with a coherent clinico-pathological correlation.

Discussion

During the triennium 1985–87 there were no deaths due to haemorrhage from placenta praevia and pre-eclampsia was not a significant feature in any of the four placental abruptions. Bleeding however continues to be a significant and often preventable cause of maternal death. Deficiencies in antenatal care were reflected in anaemic patients coming into labour, and high risk patients being booked for delivery in small units and without due regard to the special preparations recommended in the last Report for England and Wales. In two instances, patients were largely responsible for their own deaths in that they refused blood transfusion on religious grounds. It is, however, possible that more experienced supervision throughout labour, abdominal aortic compression and earlier surgical intervention might have prevented the fatal haemorrhage. Some patients obviously at risk were booked for delivery in hospitals with inadequate medical, midwifery and nursing cover and with no facilities for efficient intensive care on site. The importance of delivering such patients in fully staffed and equipped hospitals with immediately available facilities for intensive care and blood transfusion cannot be over emphasised (See Annexe, Chapter 3). Internal iliac artery ligation or hysterectomy, performed early and expertly can be life saving; the decision to adopt these extreme measures however, can be difficult and should never be left to relatively inexperienced doctors.

Resuscitation of hypovolaemic patients was frequently unsatisfactory in that the severity of the haemorrhage, because of inadequate monitoring, was not appreciated earlier, cross-matched blood was not readily available, and severely shocked patients were sometimes treated by junior anaesthetic and obstetric staff. With one exception all of these contributing causes of death from haemorrhage were considered to be preventable.

Annexe to Chapter 3

Guidelines for the management of massive obstetric haemorrhage

Summon all the extra staff required, including obstetricians, midwives and nurses. *In particular the duty anaesthetic registrar should be contacted immediately as in most obstetric units the anaesthetists will take over the management of the fluid replacement.* Alert the haematologists and the blood transfusion service who should be asked to be fully involved in the case as soon as possible. Make sure porters are available and warned that they will be required at short notice.

At least 20ml of blood should be taken (or an amount agreed by the local departments concerned) for blood grouping, cross matching and relevant coagulation studies. A minimum of six units of blood should be ordered. Whole blood is the treatment of choice. If only plasma-reduced blood is available at first, additional colloid will be necessary if more than three units of plasma-reduced blood have to be given. Human albumin solution (4.5%) is best, but degraded gelatin solutions may be more readily available and are often used in practice. Metastarch preparations may also be useful. Dextran is no longer recommended.

All patients should be given blood of their own group as soon as possible. Patients known to have anti-c antibodies from their antenatal records should not be given Group O Rh-negative blood. For other patients with severe haemorrhage, uncross-matched Group O Rh-negative blood can be life saving.

At least two peripheral infusion lines should be set up using cannulae of not less than 14 gauge. Central venous pressure (CVP) monitoring should immediately be set up since it helps ensure that therapy is safely controlled. Central venous pressure should be continuously displayed and a display of intra-arterial pressure is also extremely useful.

Facilities for the measurement and display of CVP, intra-arterial pressure, ECG, heart rate, blood gases and acid base status should be available to all consultant obstetric units.

Regular haemoglobin or haematocrit assessment can be helpful in the control of blood and fluid therapy, but restoration of normovolaemia is the first priority. Do not give fresh frozen plasma or platelet concentrates until major haemorrhage has been stopped or until approximately five units of stored blood have been given rapidly. It is a waste of these scarce materials to give them before this, particularly if there is active bleeding from a source which should be controlled by immediate surgery. Relevant coagulation studies should be carried out so that optimal replacement therapy with blood and blood products can be determined.

Rapid administration of fluids intravenously should be achieved by use of a compression cuff on the plastic bag. Martin's pumps and chambers for hand pumping do not give blood fast enough in exsanguinated patients and should not be used.

Blood must be administered through blood warming equipment.

Blood filtration is not usually necessary and may delay blood transfusion.

Additional calcium administration is rarely required and only if there is evidence of Ca deficiency. 10% calcium chloride is preferable to calcium gluconate.

All patients with prolonged or massive haemorrhage requires proper monitoring of pulse rate, blood pressure, CVP, blood gases, acid base status and urinary output as well as dedicated continuing care by the midwifery, nursing and medical staff. Early consideration should be given to the advantages of transfer to an intensive care unit.

More detailed reading

1.   British Society of Haematology Guidelines for transfusion for massive blood loss. *Clin. Lab. Haemat* 1988; 10: 265–273.
2.   Hewitt P E and Machin S J. Massive Blood Transfusion. *Brit. Med. J* 1990; 300: 107–109.

CHAPTER 4

Thrombosis and thromboembolism

Summary

There were 29 deaths from pulmonary embolism counted in this chapter. There was one death from pulmonary embolism which followed a spontaneous abortion during 1985–87, which has been counted in Chapter 6 but considered in this chapter. There was another death from widespread arterial thrombosis. There were also two deaths from sagittal sinus thrombosis which have been included in this chapter but separately described. There was another death from cerebral infarction associated with carotid artery thrombosis which is counted and described in Chapter 12.

Excluding the death from pulmonary embolism after abortion, there were 16 antepartum deaths and 14 postpartum, including the death from arterial thrombosis. Seven of the 16 antepartum deaths occurred before the 18th week and 15 before the thirty-third week. At autopsy most of the women who died antenatally had unrecognised deep venous thrombosis. In the majority of cases this diagnosis had not been considered a possibility before death, and in four in which it had, routine investigations were negative so that thromboembolism was thought to have been excluded.

Seven of the deaths from pulmonary embolism, and the death from arterial thrombosis, followed Caesarean section, and 10 of the 14 postpartum deaths occurred after discharge from hospital.

Thrombosis and thromboembolism

Deaths from thromboembolism, and sagittal sinus thrombosis are counted as Direct causes of maternal death and discussed in this chapter. Twenty nine deaths were coded as pulmonary embolism (ICD 673.2); and one other death from pulmonary embolism ten days after a spontaneous abortion (ICD 634.6) has been counted in Chapter 6 but included in the discussion and Tables on pulmonary embolism in this chapter, to make a total of 30.

One unusual case of widespread arterial thrombosis has been coded to ICD 671.8, and there was another death from cerebral infarction associated with carotid artery thrombosis counted and described in Chapter 12. Two cases were due to sagittal sinus thrombosis (ICD 671.5) Two other deaths are mentioned in this chapter but counted in Chapters 2 and 5 respectively. One, a woman who had eclampsia, died from a terminal pulmonary embolism, and a woman who died from amniotic fluid embolism also had a pulmonary embolus present.

Including both the deaths following abortion and the death from arterial thrombosis, 17 deaths (ie just over half) occurred during the antenatal period and 14 after delivery. One of the latter group also survived an antenatal pulmonary embolism and is discussed in detail later.

The 30 deaths from pulmonary embolism in the UK in 1985–87 are compared with those for England and Wales for the period 1970–87 in Table 4.1. In these Tables it has to be remembered that the cases include the woman who died following a spontaneous abortion, but the arterial thrombosis death is excluded.

Table 4.1 *Deaths from pulmonary embolism, England & Wales 1970–87, compared with United Kingdom 1985–87.*

		Deaths after abortion or ectopic pregnancy	Deaths during pregnancy	Deaths during labour	Deaths after vaginal delivery	Deaths after Caesarean section	Total
England & Wales	1970–72	10	14	—	22 (11.6)	15 (145.2)	61
	1973–75	3	14	—	13 (7.7)	6 (59.2)	36
	1976–78	2	14	—	20 (12.7)	9 (74.6)	45
	1979–81	5	1	1	4 (2.4)	7 (41.9)	28
	1982–84	4	9	—	4 (2.4)	12 (64.6)	29
	1985–87	1	16	—	5 (N/A)	3 (N/A)	25
United Kingdom	1985–87	1	16	—	6 (N/A)	7 (N/A)	30*

Rates per million vaginal deliveries or Caesarean section deliveries given in parentheses.
* Death after arterial thrombosis excluded.

It will be noted that there were more deaths prior to delivery than in any previous triennium.

A comparison of the interval between delivery and death following vaginal deliveries and Caesarean section is shown in Tables 4.2 and 4.3. The numbers are small during the period studied (1970–87) but a higher proportion of the deaths occur in the first 14 days after delivery regardless of the mode of delivery.

Table 4.2 *Interval between delivery and pulmonary embolism following vaginal delivery, England and Wales 1970–87, compared with United Kingdom 1985–87.*

		up to 7 days	8–14 days	15–42 days	Total
England & Wales	1970–87	27 (39.7%)	14 (20.6%)	27* (39.7%)	68 (100%)
United Kingdom	1985–87	—	3	3	6

* Includes one in which the time of birth was concealed by the mother but the interval based on the autopsy findings, was within 42 days.

Table 4.3 *Interval between delivery and pulmonary embolism following Caesarean section, England and Wales 1970–87, compared with United Kingdom 1985–87.*

		up to 7 days	8–14 days	15–42 days	Total
England & Wales	1970–87	19 (36.5%)	12 (23.1%)	21 (40.4%)	52 (100%)
United Kingdom	1985–87	1	2	4	7*

* Arterial thrombosis death excluded.

Antenatal deaths

An analysis of the period of gestation of all the antenatal deaths in 1985–87, including the death counted as due to spontaneous abortion, is as follows:–

Up to 12 weeks	6 deaths
13–27 weeks	4 deaths
28 weeks to term	7 deaths*

* includes a concealed pregnancy death.

The salient clinical features of these 17 deaths are given in Table 4.4. Fifteen of these women were aged 25 years and over and nine of them aged 30 years and over.

Table 4.4 *Clinical features of antenatal deaths from pulmonary embolism.*

Gestation in weeks	Features noted
6	Chest pain
7	Total bed rest for one week
7	Inpatient, psychiatric ward (counted in Chapter 6)
8	Chest pain
11	Hyperemesis, complete bed rest 3 weeks
11	Tightness in chest, dyspnoea
13	Fainting episodes
16	Inpatient 2 weeks
21	Pain in thigh (muscular)
26	(Palpitations, dyspnoea and tachycardia.
	(Cause undiagnosed.
28	Varicose veins. Sudden collapse. Postmortem CS**.
28	Chest pain, varicose veins, ligation of inferior vena cava
30	Dyspnoea, diagnosis considered. Postmortem CS**.
31	Chest pain. Undiagnosed.
32	Sudden death
37	Sudden collapse
38*	Concealed pregnancy. Sudden collapse.

* Estimated.
** CS = Caesarean section.

There were eight deaths associated with early pregnancy problems all before the 17th week of gestation. This emphasises that thromboembolism must be considered a possible diagnosis even at an early stage of pregnancy. Chest pain and dyspnoea followed by sudden collapse were the most common symptoms in antenatal patients. In only two women was the diagnosis considered and treatment commenced, albeit unsuccessfully. The diagnosis of thromboembolism was considered in three other women but dismissed because of a lack of clinical signs or negative findings so that anticoagulant therapy did not appear to have been considered in any of them. There were clinical features highly suggestive of pulmonary embolism in another two women but no diagnosis made before their sudden death.

Autopsy findings in antepartum cases

Autopsy revealed thrombosis in the pelvic or leg veins in 14 of the 16 women in whom autopsy was performed. Autopsy was refused or not performed in two instances. The left leg was involved in 10 of the 12 women where the leg veins were found to contain thrombus. Indeed in only two instances was any thrombus noted in the right leg. Thus despite the lack of clinical signs the leg veins contained thrombus in the majority of the women who died from antepartum pulmonary embolism.

One case had unusual dual pathology. This women, who actually died from widespread amniotic fluid embolism and is described in Chapter 5, also had had an unsuspected antepartum pulmonary embolism.

Two women had postmortem Caesarean sections, one baby died and the other survived but is severely disabled.

Antepartum and postpartum thromboembolism

A young multipara was admitted at 35+ weeks gestation because of several episodes of haemoptysis. No lesion was found by a physician or an ENT surgeon. A chest X-ray and Doppler examination of the leg veins were normal. An ECG showed right ventricular strain with possible pulmonary embolism. The patient, however, went home against medical advice. One week later she was readmitted with further haemoptysis. Labour was induced a few days later and she had an emergency Caesarean section because of fetal distress. She collapsed on her second postoperative day. A diagnosis of pulmonary embolism was made and intravenous heparin therapy was commenced. Despite this therapy her progress was slow. In the second postpartum week she had all the clinical features of a large pulmonary embolus and died. Permission for an autopsy was refused.

Anticoagulant therapy had not been considered antenatally on her readmission because of further haemoptysis.

Postpartum pulmonary embolism

There were 13 postpartum deaths due to pulmonary embolism including the case just described. Brief clinical details of all 13 cases are given in Table 4.5.

Postpartum pulmonary embolism and sagittal sinus thrombosis

An older parous woman had a history of deep vein thrombosis (DVT) though this had not been declared by the patient when she was seen at the booking clinic. At 37 weeks she had a forceps delivery for fetal distress. She was discharged home on the third day and readmitted a few days later for evacuation of retained products of conception and discharged the following day. She collapsed at home about a week later having had headaches and episodes of loss of consciousness. In view of her previous history of DVT a diagnosis of cortical vein thrombosis was made. After investigation, including a CT scan it was considered by a neurologist that she had suffered a small cerebral haemorrhage and therefore she did not receive anticoagulant therapy. On the 27th postpartum day she had a cardiac arrest and died.

Table 4.5 *Postpartum thromboembolism*

	Postpartum day	Mode of delivery	Features
Venous	1	CS	Fibroid and obstructed labour.
	8	ND	Sudden collapse.
	8	CS	Obese; anaemia, 3rd day 'something behind sternum and wanted to cough it up'. Chest infection diagnosed but not confirmed at autopsy.
	9	CS	Antepartum and postpartum thromboembolism (described in text).
	11	ND	Painful leg. Oral anti-inflammatory agent. Sudden collapse.
	13	ND	Dyspnoea considered due to obesity. Sudden death.
	17	CS	Wound infection and dehiscence. Sudden collapse. Post-mortem, longstanding emboli.
	19	CS	Wound infection. Chest discomfort.
	27	FD	Postpartum embolus and cerebral sinus thrombus (described in text).
	28	ND	Premature labour at 34 weeks. Sudden collapse.
	29	ND	Obese. Pain in leg. Anti-inflammatory agent. Sudden collapse.
	35	CS	Sudden collapse.
	42	CS	Antepartum haemorrhage. Flying Squad. Cerebral symptoms, ?cerebral sinus thrombosis. Sudden collapse.
Arterial	22	CS	Wound infection. Cerebral signs. Arterial embolectomy right leg.

ND = Normal delivery
FD = Forceps delivery
CS = Caesarean section

Autopsy revealed a superior sagittal sinus thrombus with no evidence of cerebral haemorrhage or infarction. Death was due to a large coiled thrombus in both main pulmonary arteries. There was thrombus in the calf veins, but not in the femoral or iliac veins.

Autopsy findings in the postpartum deaths

Autopsy was refused or not performed on two women. The site of thrombus was looked for in another two women, but not found. In the other 10 autopsies thrombus was found in the pelvic veins only in three, in the pelvic and leg veins in two, and in the leg veins only in the other five. There was no predominance of thrombus on the left side in the postpartum cases as had been noted in women who died antepartum.

Clinical features

Apart from those women who collapsed suddenly the others experienced a variety of symptoms. These included either pain or discomfort in the legs, or respiratory symptoms, mainly dyspnoea or difficulty in breathing. Two of the more unusual presentations have been described in detail.

One woman had a forceps delivery, five had normal deliveries and seven had Caesarean sections.

Arterial thrombosis

An elderly parous woman, who had her pregnancy terminated by a Caesarean section, developed a wound infection. She remained well until the 14th day when she developed right arm weakness and dysphasia. She was started on heparin and despite heparin infusion she deteriorated neurologically. The CT scan findings were in keeping with cerebral infarcts. A few days later an arterial occlusion of the right leg was treated by embolectomy. Her right leg improved initially but deteriorated in accord with her general condition and she died on the 22nd day.

The autopsy revealed widespread thrombosis within the arterial system. The right subclavian artery contained recent thrombus and the innominate artery was occluded by thrombus which had also occluded the right carotid artery. Sections of the brain showed two well defined lesions. One composed of small areas of infarcts mainly in the cerebral cortex which were of the type suggesting a period of hypovolaemic shock and the other type based on small vessels with necrosis of the wall, thrombotic occlusion and small infarcts around the vessels compatible with DIC during life.

Age

The effect of age for England and Wales for 1970–1987 inclusive is tabulated in Table 4.6. This indicates clearly that the critical age is 35 years and over. The risk being highest in women aged 40 years and over.

Table 4.6 *Maternal deaths due to pulmonary embolism by age, England and Wales 1970–87.*

Age (years)	Number	Rate per million maternities
Under 20	11	9.7
20–24	36	9.7
25–29	76	18.7
30–34	43	21.2
35–39	38	57.3
40 and over	18	123.0
All Ages	222	18.9

A similar effect is noted for the figures for the United Kingdom in 1985–87 in Table 4.7.

Substandard Care

The diagnosis of antenatal thrombosis or pulmonary embolism did not even appear to have been considered in the majority of the fatal cases which occurred during the course of pregnancy. Unless there is a high index of suspicion, the diagnosis will continue to be missed by those involved in the care of pregnant women. Pain in the chest, dyspnoea or

Table 4.7 *Maternal deaths due to pulmonary embolism by age, United Kingdom 1985–87.*

Age (years)	Number	Rate per million maternities
Under 20	1	5.2
20–24	2	3.1
25–29	13	16.7
30–34	6	13.7
35–39	6	39.4
40 and over	2	75.1
All ages	30	13.4

tachycardia should be considered the symptoms of pulmonary embolism until proved otherwise and treatment instituted on suspicion. Despite autopsy findings of deep vein thrombosis, the condition was not clinically diagnosed in any of the early or late pregnancy cases.

In this triennium, even though many postpartum deaths were sudden and unexpected, there appeared to have been sufficient warning symptoms and signs for anticoagulants to have been given. Indeed, in many instances the autopsy findings indicated that thrombosis had been present for a considerable time. Conservative measures such as anti-inflammatory agents were frequently used, although always unlikely to be effective in the treatment of deep vein thrombosis associated with pregnancy. Prophylactic anticoagulant therapy, even in high risk patients, was rarely given.

Cerebral thrombosis

There were two cases of proven sagittal sinus thrombosis.

The first case of sagittal sinus thrombosis occurred in a primigravida who was found to have antibodies present during a routine test at booking. These were later confirmed as Lupus anticoagulant. She was admitted as an emergency in mid-pregnancy because of two grand mal convulsions. The neurologists considered she had cerebral vein thrombosis and this diagnosis was supported by a CT scan. Treatment with corticosteroids and/or anticoagulant and/or antibiotics was discussed but the physicians considered that there were contraindications to each of these drugs. The agreed management was bed rest with adequate hydration. A few days later she collapsed and became deeply unconscious. A further CT scan revealed a massive largely clotted left temporal haematoma. This had ruptured through into the ventricular system and there was brain stem compression and displacement and coning at the tentorium. She died later that day. On religious grounds and because of the CT findings an autopsy was not performed.

The association of Lupus anticoagulant with a variety of thromboembolic disorders is well recognised.

The second case was that of a young multipara who had a normal delivery at term. She complained of headaches after delivery for which no cause could be found by the obstetric team. She was seen the day after her discharge from hospital by her general practitioner and an on-call doctor who found no abnormality to account for her headache. As she became more drowsy a third on-call doctor admitted her to hospital. She became comatose and a CT scan showed a probable large occipital haemorrhage. She died a day later.

A Coroner's autopsy revealed a recent thrombotic occlusion of the venous sinus of the dura mater. Detailed neuropathological examination of the brain showed well established and organised antemortem thrombus occluding the proximal part of the sagittal sinus, together with the adjacent transverse sinuses and inferior sagittal sinus. More distally the superior sagittal sinus was also occluded by more recent looking thrombus. There was also thrombosis of parasagittal bridging veins draining into the superior sagittal sinus. The appearances suggested propagation of clots anteriorly along the superior sagittal sinus. All this had resulted in extensive bilateral infarction of the cerebral hemispheres with concomitant brain swelling and tentorial and tonsillar herniation.

Discussion

Venous thromboembolism is the major cause of maternal death in the United Kingdom. Unfortunately there apparently remains a reluctance to consider it as a possible diagnosis during pregnancy and, particularly, in early pregnancy. The majority of the women who died had no clinical evidence of deep venous thrombosis yet autopsy revealed thrombosis in the pelvic and leg veins. The potential dangers of anticoagulant therapy producing antepartum or postpartum bleeding appear to have been exaggerated. Chest X-Rays, ECG or blood gases not in keeping with the diagnosis of pulmonary embolism were the principal reasons for not giving treatment, despite the presence of one or more of the following:— dyspnoea, chest pain, hyperventilation or cyanosis. Chest infection was usually considered the more likely diagnosis in the absence of clinically detectable deep vein thrombosis. The finding of thrombosis in the majority of autopsies emphasises the unreliability of the clinical signs of deep vein thrombosis. Antibiotic and anticoagulant therapy given together might have prevented death from pulmonary embolism.

We are still unable to assess whether the use of subcutaneous heparin or anti-thromboembolic stockings has influenced the number of deaths. At present we have no idea of how frequently they are used. We are aware that the calf veins of women being delivered by Caesarean section are often nowadays protected yet it must be stressed that the majority of the postnatal women who died from pulmonary embolism regardless of the mode of their delivery had been discharged at the usual time from hospital and were fairly mobile. Obesity was reported in many of the autopsies but we have been unable to compare the weight at death with the preconception or booking weight.

At the present time our recommendations must be that any woman who is pregnant or has recently been pregnant and has a suspected deep vein thrombosis or pulmonary embolism should be given full heparin anti-coagulant therapy. If postpartum, then a bilateral venogram and lung scan should be carried out within 24–48 hours. The subsequent management can then be based on the precise site of the thrombus and any evidence of embolisation.

Whilst venograms are contraindicated in the first trimester of pregnancy, even though the uterus can be shielded off, they can certainly be used in the third, and possibly the second, trimester. If real time ultrasound scanning is available this can be used in pregnancy even though it is unlikely to detect thrombus in the iliac veins because of the gravid uterus. In these circumstances it is unlikely that there will be significant thrombus in the iliac veins without there also being some in the femoral veins, a fact confirmed in the autopsies in this triennium. A ventilation-perfusion isotope lung scan can be used for the diagnosis of pulmonary embolism as the radiation dosage to the fetus is low, certainly less than that of X-ray pelvimetry. Whilst risk factors were identified in the previous England and Wales reports (Table 4.8) there still appeared in 1985–1987 to be a reluctance to use prophylactic anticoagulants in high risk patients. This particularly applied to those involved in contact with a woman at home after delivery.

Table 4.8 *Risk factors for development of thromboembolism*

Previous thromboembolism
Obesity
Immobilisation
Operative delivery
Lupus anticoagulant

Just as antepartum haemorrhage is considered to be due to placenta praevia until proved otherwise, all those looking after or involved in the care of pregnant or recently pregnant women should consider pain in the leg, pain in the chest, or dyspnoea in an otherwise healthy woman to be due to thrombosis or pulmonary embolism until proved otherwise, and ensure that the appropriate treatment is instituted. Following this the onus is to confirm, or refute, the diagnosis as soon as possible.

CHAPTER 5

Amniotic Fluid Embolism

Summary

There were nine proven deaths due to amniotic fluid embolism in the United Kingdom (UK) in 1985–87 compared with 14 in England and Wales in 1982–84. Amniotic fluid embolism was present in two other deaths, due to ruptured uterus.

The age, parity, mode of delivery, use of oxytocic drugs for augmentation of labour and presenting symptoms have been reviewed, but no specific aetiological factors were identified.

It is recommended that all women who initially survive for a few days in an intensive care unit should have their pelvic and uterine vasculature examined carefully at autopsy for the presence of any amniotic fluid material.

Amniotic fluid embolism

Only deaths where autopsy provided conclusive proof of amniotic fluid embolism have been accepted for the UK report for 1985–87. Amniotic fluid embolism was present in two other Direct deaths but not considered to be the prime cause of death. The reason for classifying the principal cause of death as ruptured uterus in these cases is discussed in this chapter as well as in Chapter 8.

There were nine Direct deaths attributed to amniotic fluid embolism and classified under ICD 673.1. There were two deaths in which there was a clinical impression of amniotic fluid embolism but no evidence of amniotic fluid in the circulation was found despite careful and detailed autopsies. Both cases are counted in Chapter 10, and are classified as sudden deaths of unknown cause. One occurring in labour and one immediately postpartum.

Age

Table 5.1 gives details of the age of the women with proven amniotic fluid embolism for England and Wales inclusive.

Table 5.2 shows the number of deaths from histologically confirmed amniotic fluid embolism for England and Wales for the triennia 1970–87 compared with the cases found in 1985–87 in England and Wales and in the UK. There were two cases** in this triennium where there were clinical

Table 5.1 *All maternal deaths with amniotic fluid embolism present by age and estimated rates per million maternities, England & Wales 1970–87.*

Age (years)	Number	Rate per million maternities
Under 20	3	2.6
20–24	15	4.0
25–29	20	4.9
30–34	21	10.4
35–39	18	27.1
40 and over	7	47.8
All ages	84	7.1

Table 5.2 *Deaths from amniotic fluid embolism histologically confirmed and deaths suspected of being amniotic fluid embolism but not confirmed, England and Wales 1970–87, compared with United Kingdom 1985–87.*

	Histologically confirmed cases	Suspected cases
1970–72	14 (2)	8
1973–75	14 (1)	7
1976–78	11 (–)	8
1979–81	18 (–)	6
1982–84	14 (1)	2
1985–87	9 (2)	1**
1985–87*	9 (2)	2**

The numbers in parentheses ( ) are with amniotic fluid embolism present but attributable to other Direct cause.
* United Kingdom data.
** See text.

features suggestive of amniotic fluid embolism even though in one case the fetal sac was intact at delivery. Although the diagnosis was positively excluded at autopsy, they have been classified as 'suspected cases', and included in Table 5.2 for comparison with previous triennia. Although the greater awareness by pathologists of this condition as a cause of maternal death during or immediately following labour makes it easier to exclude this condition there still remains a hard core of unexplained sudden deaths. They are, as already mentioned, counted in Chapter 10.

Clinical features

Table 5.3 classifies the time interval from the first symptoms or collapse till death as rapid, despite resuscitative measures, and those in whom death due to amniotic fluid embolism was relatively delayed.

Only two of the six women, whose deaths occurred within a short time of the first symptoms of collapse, had disseminated intravascular co-agulation (DIC). In one of these women it was an autopsy and not a clinical finding. In all three women where death was delayed DIC was clinically present.

Table 5.3 *Oxytocic agents and disseminated intravascular coagulation in amniotic fluid embolism cases.*

Collapse to death	Oxytocic	Disseminated intravascular coagulation
Rapid	Prostaglandin pessary (× 2)	No
Rapid	—	No
Rapid	—	No
Rapid	Prostaglandin pessary	Yes
Rapid	—	No
Rapid	*Syntocinon* bolus given I.V. in 3rd stage.	Yes
Slow	Prostaglandin pessary	Yes
Slow	*Syntocinon* infusion	Yes
Slow	*Syntocinon* infusion	Yes

Six of the nine women had received Prostaglandin or *Syntocinon*. Uterine contractions were noted to be strong in five and fetal distress was noted in the other. One woman with an intrauterine death in a concealed pregnancy, collapsed and died shortly after admission in labour.

Symptoms

Analysis of the presenting symptoms, stage of labour and action regarding delivery for the nine women detailed in Table 5.3 is given in Table 5.4

Table 5.4 *Clinical features of deaths from amniotic fluid embolism*.*

Stage of labour	Action regarding delivery	Symptoms
First (premature labour)	CS** after death	Nauseated, dyspnoea, central cyanosis.
First	Emergency CS**	Grand mal fit, cardiac arrest.
First	CS** after death	Said 'something wrong with my heart' 5 minutes before became unconscious.
First	Undelivered	Fit, cardiac arrest and DIC.
First	Undelivered	Concealed pregnancy. Cyanosed and incoherent.
Third	Elective CS**	Asthmatic. Tightness of chest, dyspnoea.
First	Emergency CS**	Dyspnoea, semi-conscious and centrally cyanosed followed by DIC.
Third/postpartum	Forceps delivery	DIC. 3 hours later bronchospasm prior to collapse.
Third/postpartum	Forceps delivery	Dyspnoea. DIC. Resuscitation. ITU care. Died 8th day, ARDS†.

*   Cases are listed in the same order as in Table 5.3
** CS — Caesarean section.
† ARDS — Adult respiratory distress syndrome.

Dyspnoea and central cyanosis were the principal symptoms and signs in the majority of women. The presenting feature in two cases was a fit. The death of the first six cases detailed in Table 5.3 and 5.4 occurred within

30 minutes of the first symptoms or signs. This might reflect the volume of amniotic fluid material which entered the circulation or the degree of reaction to it. One woman survived 8 days in an intensive care unit (ICU) having had a hysterectomy because of DIC. Extensive evidence of material from amniotic fluid was present in the uterine vasculature, thus confirming the diagnosis which would have been missed if the hysterectomy specimen had not been examined in detail. The autopsy revealed typical features of the adult respiratory distress syndrome (ARDS) but no amniotic squames were identified in the lungs after a thorough search by an experienced obstetrical pathologist. The absence of amniotic squames in the lungs was attributed to their disappearance from the pulmonary circulation during the 8 days of survival in the ICU.

Undelivered

One woman, with an intrauterine death and who died undelivered, had concealed her pregnancy. The other woman who died undelivered collapsed and died 10 minutes after surgical rupture of membranes at 4 cm dilatation.

Mode of delivery

Forceps

One woman had a forceps delivery carried out after a protracted labour in which an oxytocic infusion was administered for over 12 hours.

Another woman, who had severely diminished respiratory function, had a prophylactic forceps delivery because of marked respiratory distress, developed DIC and had a hysterectomy. She survived for eight days in an ICU.

Caesarean section

One woman who had an elective Caesarean section was a severe asthmatic. She was given an intravenous bolus dose of *Syntocinon* as her baby was delivered. Almost immediately afterwards she collapsed and died suddenly.

The two emergency Caesarean sections were carried out for fetal distress which in both cases occurred immediately following artificial rupture of the membranes.

The two postmortem Caesarean sections were carried out after the mothers had suddenly collapsed and died in labour. Both babies were stillborn.

In only one of the nine women was there a comment about a possible excess of amniotic fluid. She had a controlled ARM done 45 minutes before she had difficulty in breathing.

Autopsies

The diagnosis was confirmed by examination of the lungs in all but one case. In the latter case, a woman who survived 8 days in an ICU before dying from ARDS, the vasculature of the uterus removed by hysterectomy showed amniotic squames.

A tear in the cervix was reported in one case.

One autopsy revealed thrombus in the right pelvic veins and an occlusive thromboembolus in a major branch of the pulmonary artery.

The combination of thromboembolism and amniotic fluid embolism is very unusual.

Other Direct deaths and amniotic fluid embolism

There were two Direct deaths attributed to rupture of the uterus. One had a complete but undiagnosed rupture and the other an incomplete rupture. In both rupture was considered to have preceded the injection of amniotic fluid into the circulation. They are both discussed in detail in Chapter 8.

Substandard care

In no case was there evidence of substandard medical care. One women whose fetus had died in-utero was considered to have contributed to her own death by concealing her pregnancy.

Pathology

All nine cases came to autopsy. Details are shown in Table 16.1. One autopsy report was considered to be substandard because of the description of the postmortem findings. In all but one of the cases there was histological confirmation of amniotic fluid in the maternal circulation. This was provided by examination of the pulmonary vasculature alone in four cases (one only by frozen section at the time of autopsy). In one case amniotic squames were demonstrated only in the hysterectomy specimen.

Discussion

The characteristic clinical features of amniotic fluid embolism are sudden dyspnoea, hypoxia and hypotension. These features may be followed in minutes by cardio-respiratory arrest. In some cases grand mal seizures accompany the initial clinical events. An element of ARDS may be present. A haemorrhagic phase may accompany the initial haemodynamic disturbances or follow them if the woman survives the initial phase. No relationship has ever been demonstrated between the severity of the clinical features and the amount of particulate material in the lungs. This lack of correlation may reflect the degree of reaction to particular components of amniotic fluid rather than the quantity entering the circulation.

As in the past, analysis of fatal cases of amniotic fluid embolism in this enquiry has not revealed specific aetiological factors. It is not known whether amniotic fluid can enter the maternal circulation, like fetal red cells under certain circumstances, without producing serious side-effects. Non-fatal cases have been reported, but a conclusive test for amniotic fluid embolism comparable to the Kleihauer test for the presence of fetal cells in the maternal circulation, is not available.

Our insistence on positive proof of amniotic fluid embolism has resulted in cases of sudden death often suspected as due to amniotic fluid embolism being identified and classified to other Direct causes. In 1985–87 confirmed amniotic fluid embolism in the pulmonary circulation was found in two women with ruptured uterus whose deaths are counted in Chapter 8.

All three of the women who survived for more than 30 minutes developed typical clinical features of DIC compared with only one out of six women who died suddenly after the first symptoms of collapse.

Since 1970, the Confidential Enquiries for England and Wales have noted possible risk factors in women who died from amniotic fluid embolism. They include age over 35 years, high parity, excessive or strong uterine contractions, the use of oxytocic drugs for induction or augmentation of labour, and, in particular, a single bolus dose of *Syntocinon* or *Syntometrine*, overdistension of the uterus, complete or incomplete rupture of the uterus and intravascular coagulation. One or more of these factors were present in each of the nine deaths. However, the majority of women who have one or more of these factors present do not die in labour from amniotic fluid embolism. The purpose of mentioning these features is to stress that extra care may be appropriate for the women who have one or more of them.

It will be noted from a comparison of the number of cases which were reported for England and Wales, 14 (1973–75), 11 (1976–78), 18 (1979–81) and 14 (1982–84), that the number of histologically confirmed amniotic fluid deaths has fallen in this triennium especially as cases from Scotland and Northern Ireland in 1985–87 are now included. Whether this is due to chance or reflects greater care in the management of labour in general only future reports will show.

CHAPTER 6

Early pregnancy deaths (including abortion)

Summary

All deaths from ectopic pregnancy and abortion have been aggregated under the heading of Early Pregnancy Deaths, including two after 28 weeks of gestation in abdominal ectopic pregnancies.

There were 36 deaths in early pregnancy in this triennium. Twenty two were Direct deaths, of which 16 were due to ectopic pregnancy, four to spontaneous abortion, one to ruptured uterus with missed abortion and one to legal abortion. Of the remaining 14 deaths not counted in this chapter, 12 were in women who had a spontaneous abortion and two in women whose pregnancies had been terminated. No deaths were ascribed to illegal abortion.

Substandard care was considered to have contributed to death in seven of the Direct deaths from ectopic pregnancy, and in none of the women dying from spontaneous or legal abortion.

The number of deaths from ectopic pregnancy and spontaneous abortion is similar to that previously reported for England and Wales. Due to the lack of suitable data it has not been possible to calculate the rates relative to all ectopic pregnancies or to the number of estimated pregnancies (Table 6.1).

Ectopic pregnancy

Ectopic pregnancy accounted for 9.1% of all Direct maternal deaths in this triennium. There were 11 deaths in England and Wales, which is similar to the number (10) in the previous triennium. In addition a further five women died from this cause elsewhere in the United Kingdom in this triennium, making a total of 16. Fifteen deaths were coded to ICD 633 and one, which was complicated by sepsis, to ICD 639. Data relating age and parity to the deaths are not available for ectopic pregnancy.

Details of the 16 women dying from ectopic pregnancy are given in Table 6.2. There were 14 cases of tubal pregnancy and two cases of abdominal pregnancy. There was a history of tubal damage or abnormality in seven cases. In seven cases there was a history of substandard care and these cases are described.

A young woman known to be pregnant started to bleed heavily at nine weeks gestation, and was diagnosed as having a threatened abortion by

Table 6.1 *Deaths from ectopic pregnancies and rates per million estimated pregnancies, England and Wales 1970–87 compared with United Kingdom 1985–87.* *

	Triennium	Total estimated pregnancies*	Ectopic pregnancies* in HIPE†	Ectopic pregnancies per 10,000 estimated pregnancies	Number of deaths	Deaths per million estimated pregnancies	Deaths per 1,000 ectopic pregnancies
England and Wales	1970–72	2,890.7	11.6	40	34	11.8	2.9
	1973–75	2,578.4	11.7	45	19	7.4	1.6
	1976–78	2,323.0	11.6	50	21	9.0	1.8
	1979–81	2,543.2	12.1	48	20	7.9	1.7
	1982–84	2,507.0	14.4	57	10**	4.0	0.7
	1985–87	2,650.9	N/A	N/A	11	4.1	N/A
United Kingdom	1985–87	N/A	N/A	N/A	16	N/A	N/A

* In thousands
** There were 3 other deaths from anaesthesia
† HIPE — Hospital In-patient Enquiry

Table 6.2 *Summary of details of women dying from ectopic pregnancy United Kingdom 1985–87.*

Trimester	Past history of tubal damage	Site of ectopic pregnancy	Substandard care
Unknown	No	Tube	No
First	No	Tube	Yes
First	No	Tube	Yes
First	No	Tube	No
First	No	Tube	Yes
First	PID	Tube	No
First	PID	Tube	Yes
First	No	Tube	Yes
First	No	Tube	No
First	Sterilised	Tube	Yes
First	Caesarean section × 2	Tube	No
Second	Uterine	Tube abnormality	No
Second	No	Cornu	No
First	PID	Cornu	No
Third	No	Abdominal	No
Third	PID	Abdominal	Yes

(PID — History of pelvic inflammatory disease)

her general practitioner. An ultrasound scan was considered but not carried out, nor is there evidence of a vaginal examination having been done. She was seen by her general practitioner a few days later with severe abdominal pain, vomiting and further vaginal bleeding. A diagnosis of gastroenteritis was made but shortly afterwards she collapsed and died. The autopsy revealed a ruptured right tubal pregnancy.

The exact details of this case are obscured because this general practitioner's notes were destroyed three years after the patient's death, in conformity with local family Practitioner Committee practice.

The second case concerns a woman with a long history of primary infertility who at eight weeks of pregnancy came to a casualty department with vaginal bleeding. Despite the finding of a positive pregnancy test and an empty uterus on ultrasound scan she was sent home. She was admitted three days later complaining of lower abdominal pain and vomiting. The following day the abdominal pain was still present with a tachycardia and eventually she fainted. She was seen twice by a senior house officer (SHO) who failed to appreciate the significance of the symptoms and signs. Six hours after the doctor's last visit the patient was found unconscious and died. Autopsy revealed a ruptured right tubal pregnancy.

The third case concerns a woman admitted to a surgical unit with a history of several laparotomies for a gangrenous bowel, who now had severe abdominal pain. She had had regular periods until one month before, since when she had had irregular vaginal bleeding. On admission she was found to have a haemoglobin concentration of 4.2g/dl. She was seen by a gynaecologist who could find no evidence of gynaecological pathology and who did not suspect pregnancy. Although he advised an ultrasound scan on the following day no record of the result is available. Despite transfusion with 6 units of blood she collapsed 48 hours later.

An emergency operation revealed a ruptured tubal pregnancy and several holes in the small intestine for which there was no obvious cause. The tube was removed and the holes in the intestine were repaired. The intra-abdominal bleeding persisted, so that a further laparotomy was done at which no new bleeding points were found. The patient never regained consciousness and died shortly afterwards.

The fourth case was a young woman who collapsed whilst visiting friends. Despite the rapid arrival of an ambulance following a '999' call, she refused to go to hospital until the local general practitioner arrived. By this time it was too late and she died before reaching hospital. The autopsy revealed a ruptured right tubal pregnancy.

The fifth case concerned a woman admitted to hospital with a classical history of an early tubal pregnancy which had ruptured. The preoperative haemoglobin concentration was 4.6g/dl. A locum registrar did a salpingectomy supervised by his consultant who considered the operation to have been well done. During the operation the blood loss was estimated to be three litres followed by a further loss of 1.4 litres postoperatively. The patient suddenly developed acute pulmonary oedema during surgery and again in the immediate postoperative period. No consideration was given to a further laparotomy. At autopsy the abdomen was full of blood and a defect was found in the broad ligament just below the site of removal of the affected tube, through which blood could be seen oozing from underlying vessels.

Central venous pressure monitoring was not used until after surgery when pulmonary oedema had already occurred. In view of the rapid onset of pulmonary oedema and the considerable amount of fluid given intravenously postoperatively it seems likely that the cause of death was circulatory overload.

The sixth case concerns a woman who had been sterilised, following which she had had intermittent pelvic pain for which no cause could be found. She was first seen by a consultant obstetrician when she was admitted to hospital as an emergency complaining of abdominal pain with what appeared to be a uterus equivalent in size to 24 weeks gestation. However an ultrasound scan revealed a fetus of only 12 weeks size with a mass apparently involving the lower uterus, thought to be a fibroid. As there was no abdominal tenderness on palpation and the patient wished to continue the pregnancy she was sent home with a diagnosis of possible degeneration in a fibroid. One week later she was readmitted in a collapsed condition and died shortly afterwards. The autopsy revealed the right tube entering a secondary abdominal pregnancy with a mass of placenta, blood clot and a fetal sac. There was evidence of bleeding from this site about a week old in addition to a large volume of fresh clot.

The last case involved a woman with a history of ulcerative colitis who had had an ileostomy following a total colectomy. Laparoscopy, as part of an investigation for infertility, had revealed a pelvis full of adhesions, and she had been told that she was certainly infertile. She therefore used no contraception. Despite three months of amenorrhoea, pregnancy was not suspected when she was admitted under the care of the surgeons having had a massive haemorrhage through her ileostomy. It was only after a further four weeks that the pregnancy was detected when barium studies were planned to investigate the cause of the bleeding, and she was then referred to an obstetrician. The fundal height was 21 cms, which agreed with her dates, but an ultrasound scan report commented on the presence of 'severe oligohydramnios'. At 32 weeks she was treated with antibiotics for repeated rigors, and a surgical opinion was requested. A week later, because of her deteriorating condition, a laparotomy was done which revealed an abdominal pregnancy with erosion of the placenta into the small bowel. The placenta was removed and the defect in the small bowel oversewn. Postoperatively she developed disseminated intravascular coagulation (DIC) and the adult respiratory distress syndrome (ARDS) associated with *Cl. Perfringens* septicaemia, from which she eventually died.

Substandard care

Care was considered to have been substandard in seven of the 16 women who died from ectopic pregnancy. Delay in making the diagnosis was again a major factor. In one case vaginal bleeding and lower abdominal pain was thought to be due to a threatened abortion without a vaginal examination being done. In several cases an ultrasound scan, which would have been critical in making the diagnosis, was omitted. In a further case, despite a positive pregnancy test and a definite ultrasound scan report that the cavity of the uterus was empty, a woman was sent home from the casualty department. In two cases clear evidence of intra-abdominal bleeding was missed. In one of these cases the presence of surgical pathology involving the bowel undoubtedly misled the gynaecologist. In one case massive fluid replacement after an operation for ectopic pregnancy led to pulmonary oedema from circulatory overload. A central venous pressure line was put up too late and the abdomen was not reopened despite evidence of continued concealed blood loss. Finally in one case the patient contributed to her own death by refusing to go to hospital until it was too late despite being severely shocked due to bleeding from a ruptured ectopic pregnancy.

Late diagnosis of an abdominal pregnancy cannot be regarded as substandard because the condition is uncommon. Nevertheless in the presence of unexplained severe abdominal pain in a woman who is known to be pregnant the possibility of this diagnosis must be borne in mind. Most obstetricians have little experience of managing these cases so that it is worthwhile mentioning that, in general, when a placenta is implanted in the abdominal cavity no attempt should be made to remove it, and the abdomen can be closed without an increased risk of secondary haemorrhage.

Discussion

Deaths from ectopic pregnancy which could possibly have been avoided continue to occur. Intra-abdominal bleeding from an ectopic pregnancy is one of the most acute and dangerous emergencies with which any doctor has to deal. It is often heralded by premonitory 'leaking' of blood before the final rupture leading to haemorrhage, which occasionally may be so severe that there is little time to stop it becoming fatal. It is in this premonitory phase that a doctor has to call on all his clinical skills in order to make the diagnosis. Modern technology has now enabled the diagnosis to be made much earlier and more exactly than in the past. In the last report we commented on the importance of using the rapid beta-hCG test to make a diagnosis of early pregnancy. Laparoscopy and ultrasound scanning are also available in all hospitals, and there is little doubt that if they had been used in some of the cases described in this report, death could have been avoided.

Probably the most important contribution to reducing the risk of death from ectopic pregnancy is an awareness by medical attendants that in any woman of reproductive age, an ectopic pregnancy may be the cause of a lower abdominal pain particularly when of sudden onset.

When a woman presents with unexplained abdominal pain with or without vaginal bleeding she should not be allowed home until every means available has been used to exclude an ectopic pregnancy. The ready availability of beta-hCG kits for the detection of early pregnancy means that general practitioners in the home or surgery can easily make a diagnosis at an early stage of pregnancy. Vaginal examination is also essential to determine whether there is localised tenderness, or a palpable appendage mass. If there is any doubt, referral to hospital is preferable to a 'wait and see' policy. Laparoscopy remains the cornerstone for investigating the possibility of an ectopic pregnancy and this should be done on any woman found to have a positive pregnancy test with an empty uterine cavity on ultrasound scan. Alternatively, if the pain persists for more than 24 hours despite a negative beta-hCG pregnancy test, then a laparoscopy should be done.

Ultrasound scanning makes an important contribution to the detection of an ectopic pregnancy but there are, at present, certain limitations to its use in this respect. The visualisation of a sac in the uterine cavity is valuable for it virtually excludes the possibility of an ectopic pregnancy except in the rare event of simultaneous extra- and intrauterine pregnancies. However it is not possible with present day equipment to visualise reliably a gestation sac in utero of gestational age less than six weeks. Equally, no reliance can be placed on the absence of an extrauterine swelling on ultrasound scan. The expertise of those doing the scan is also very variable, and it is essential that an experienced sonographer should be asked to do the scan and unsupervised occasional sonographers should be discouraged. Probably the greatest limitation to using ultrasound in the immediate diagnosis of an ectopic pregnancy is the lack of availability of a service at night. These comments should not be interpreted as dismissive of ultrasound which is a valuable aid in the diagnosis of ectopic pregnancy, but more as a recommendation for greater discrimination in its use and interpretation.

We have reported two deaths due to the dangerous condition of abdominal pregnancy. In each of them the common error was made of failing to consider such a diagnosis. A history of intermittent attacks of abdominal pain is typical. It should also be possible to reveal by ultrasound the small uterus separate from the abdominal mass. Unfortunately the condition is so uncommon that those who do the scan rarely consider the diagnosis.

Full information on one of the women described in this chapter was lacking because her general practitioner antenatal records had been sent to the local Family Practitioner Committee after her death, and destroyed after three years, in accordance with the normal practice. In this case we were concerned that so much time had elapsed before the initiation of the MCW97 report. It should be the responsibility of any doctor who knows of a maternal death to make sure that the District Medical Officer or Director of Public Health has been informed, so that the enquiries can be started as soon as possible. This is particularly important when the maternal death has occurred outside the obstetric unit, in another ward of the hospital or at home, when the necessity of reporting the death to the Confidential Enquiry may be overlooked.

Abortion

Table 6.3 contains data on the number of deaths from spontaneous, legal, illegal and unspecified abortions for succeeding triennia in England and Wales from 1970. Figures are also available for this triennium for the UK, but the rate per million pregnancies is not available. The figures show (i) no change in deaths from spontaneous abortion, (ii) a considerable fall in deaths due to legal abortion from seven (1982–84) to one (1985–87), (iii) a continuation from the last triennium of the disappearance of illegal abortion as a cause of death.

Table 6.3 *Direct abortion deaths in the triennial reports 1970–87 by type of abortion with rates per million maternities and rates per million estimated pregnancies.*

		Spontaneous	Legal	Illegal	Unspecified	Total	Rates per million maternities	Rates per million estimated pregnancies
England & Wales	1970–72	6	30[1]	37	—	73	31.8	25.3
	1973–75	4	13[2]	10	—	27	14.1	10.5
	1976–78	2[3]	8[3]	4	—	14	8.0	6.0
	1979–81	6[6]	5[4]	1	2	14	7.3	5.5
	1982–84	4[5]	7[5]	0	—	11	5.8	4.4
	1985–87	4[7]	1[8]	0	—	5	2.5	1.9
United Kingdom	1985–87	5[7]	1[8]	0	0	6	2.7	N/A

1. Does not include 7 anaesthetic deaths associated with legal abortion.
2. Does not include 1 anaesthetic death associated with legal abortion.
3. Does not include 5 anaesthetic deaths, 4 associated with legal and 1 with spontaneous abortion.
4. Does not include 1 anaesthetic death associated with legal abortion.
5. Does not include 2 anaesthetic deaths, 1 associated with legal and 1 with spontaneous abortion.
6. One other death is known to have followed a spontaneous abortion in the 1979–81 triennium but it was reported too late to be included in the Enquiry.
7. Includes one death from missed abortion.
8. Does not include 1 unexplained death associated with legal abortion.
1–8. These cases are identified in the individual types of abortion but not in the totals and rates.

Table 6.4 relates the number of spontaneous legal and illegal abortions to age using combined data from 1970–87 for England and Wales. The likely change in age and the techniques of abortion over this period mean that interpretation of the data can only be tentative. However figures on all legal abortions performed show that there is relatively little change in the age distribution. Table 6.4 shows that 30% of women who died were aged less than 25 years. The increased risk to women aged 35 years or more is revealed by the fact that 47% of those who died were in this age-group as compared with only 12–16% of all women having a legal abortion.

Table 6.4 *Number of women in the enquiry who died from abortion in England and Wales 1970–87.*

Age (Years)	Spontaneous and other abortions	Legal abortions (%)	Illegal abortions	All abortions
Under 25	11	19 (30)	21	51
25–34	7	15 (23)	23	45
35 and over	11	30 (47)	8	49
All ages	29	64 (100)	52	145

Table 6.5 shows the distribution of women who died from the various types of abortion between 1970–87 in England and Wales. Unfortunately the significance of this data cannot be reliably determined because of the considerable increase in recent years in the number of unmarried women, and the difficulty of distinguishing those who are unsupported and hence comparable to unmarried women in previous reports, from those who are in stable cohabitation whose numbers have increased in recent years.

Table 6.5 *Marital status of women who died from legal and spontaneous abortion in England and Wales 1970–87.*

	Spontaneous abortions	Unspecified abortions	Legal abortions	Illegal abortions	Total	% of all abortions
Married	24*	3	43	31	101*	70 (87)
Single, divorced or widowed	2	—	21	21	44	30 (13)
Total	26*	3	64	52	145*	100 (100)

* Includes one case of separated.
Figures in parentheses refer to distribution of married and unmarried women aged 16–44 years for all maternities during this period.

Spontaneous abortion

In this triennium there were five Direct deaths due to spontaneous abortion at 6, 10, 25, 26 and 27 weeks of pregnancy. In none of them was there evidence of substandard care.

A woman was admitted to hospital in severe shock which was thought to be due to a septic incomplete abortion. She died eleven hours later. There are no records of the care she received after admission to hospital but the fact that she was in an intensive care unit suggests she was seriously ill. This was a woman who clearly did not make use of the NHS services to get to hospital earlier and it is possible that there was criminal interference in her pregnancy.

A woman had a pulmonary embolus shortly after an evacuation of retained products.

A woman died from an air embolism during manual removal of what subsequently proved to be a placenta accreta.

A highly parous woman, who was 24 weeks pregnant, was admitted as an emergency with severe asthma and subsequently developed ARDS. Two days later she had a spontaneous abortion resulting in circulatory collapse from which she never recovered despite full and adequate treatment. She died about three weeks later having developed DIC, hepatic dysfunction, acute renal failure and pancreatitis.

Missed abortion and ruptured uterus

A woman had a huge uterine scar involving two-thirds of the anterior and one third of the posterior wall as a result of previous perforation at the time of a suction evacuation. Subsequent investigations had suggested that both tubes were blocked. The patient was advised against becoming pregnant again but was reassured that this could not occur as she was sterile. Some years later she became pregnant and was admitted at about the 26th week of pregnancy with a short history of an offensive vaginal discharge. She was found at laparotomy to have a ruptured uterus and *E. Coli* peritonitis; a subtotal hysterectomy was performed but she died shortly afterwards.

Indirect deaths

There were seven Indirect deaths associated with spontaneous abortion. There was no case of substandard care. Details of these cases are given in Table 6.6

Table 6.6 *Indirect deaths associated with spontaneous abortion.*

No.	Gestation (weeks)	Associated condition	Cause of death
1.	16	Hepatitis B	Liver failure
2.	7	Acute pyelonephritis	DIC and septicaemia
3.	21	Congenital heart disease. Infective endocarditis	Death during surgery
4.	20	Endotoxic shock	Myocarditis
5.	?	Drug abuse	Suicide
6.	16	Streptococcal pharyngitis	Septicaemia
7.	?	Alcoholism	?Cardiomyopathy

Legal abortion

There were two deaths of women who had a legal abortion.

The only Direct death counted in this chapter followed legal abortion by suction at 10 weeks gestation. Immediately after the procedure the patient became cyanosed and failed to respond to 100% oxygen or emergency cardiac resuscitatory measures. At autopsy a diagnosis of air embolism was made. The procedure appears to have been carried out correctly and there was no evidence of malfunction of the suction equipment.

The other case, who collapsed and died suddenly after the completion of the operation without any obvious cause for death being found at autopsy, is counted in Chapter 10, and is also discussed in Chapter 9.

Facilities available for cases of legal abortion.

In this triennium there were no deaths in the UK from legal abortion due to haemorrhage, compared with three deaths from this cause in England and Wales in 1982–84. However, as a reminder that all obstetric and gynaecological units should have an assured supply of blood and blood substitutes for administration in an emergency, as is required for places approved by the Secretary of State under the Abortion Act (1967), the 'Guidelines for Emergency Blood Cover' are attached as an Annex to this chapter.

Annexe to Chapter 6

Guidelines for emergency blood cover at nursing homes and private hospitals approved for abortion by the Secretary of State.

One of the requirements for places to be approved under the Abortion Act (1967) is that proper arrangements have been made to deal with any emergencies arising in the treatment of patients for termination of pregnancy. A very important part of these arrangements is the emergency provision of blood, blood products and other replacement fluids and the availability of the necessary blood tests before operations. The following guidelines (revised in 1989) represent the minimum standard of emergency blood cover acceptable to the Department of Health in England. (Similar, but not identical, guidelines are in use in Wales and Scotland. The Abortion Act does not extend to Northern Ireland.)

Revised Guidelines for routine blood testing and emergency blood cover for nursing homes and private hospitals approved for abortion by the Secretary of State

I. *Pre-operative routine blood testing for abortion patients*

1. *All patients* to be tested and the results to be available at the nursing home or hospital before operation:–
  a. Haemoglobin.
  b. Blood Group (A, B, O and Rhesus (D))
  c. Screen for atypical *red cell antibodies*.

2. *All patients*. The blood group to be performed and a sample of serum held in advance, by the hospital blood bank or private laboratory which can provide a 24-hour service for cross-matching if required.

Note Facilities should be available to enable screening for such conditions as sickle-cell disorders to be performed where indicated.

II. *Blood supplies and other IV fluids required in an emergency*

1. *Available immediately at the nursing home or hospital*
  a. Plasma protein fraction (Minimum 2 units of 500 ml)
  or Albumin 4/5%   (Minimum 2 units of 500 ml)

  Plasma protein substitute (minimum 4 litres)

  Crystalloid IV solutions (including dextrose saline and electrolyte solutions)

2. *Available immediately or within 15 minutes or requirement*

b.i *For all cases*
Either, two units of O Rhesus-negative blood to be available for use within 15 minutes (either held at the nursing home or hospital or 'earmarked' for them and held in an adjacent hospital blood bank or private laboratory);

Or If two units of O Rhesus-negative blood cannot be guaranteed within 15 minutes, two units of blood to be cross-matched in advance, *before the operation* is performed.

ii *For all cases*, found on screening to have atypical *red cell antibodies*, two units of blood to be cross-matched in advance *before the operation* is performed.

3. *Available if the emergency continues*

a. Supplies of crossmatched blood should be 'rapidly obtainable' in an emergency (not more than 60 minutes). This time should take into account geographical distance and travelling conditions at the busiest times of the day.

b. As described in Section I (2) *in all cases* serum should be held in advance at the hospital blood bank or private laboratory for cross matching if required.

4. If the emergency blood supplies available at the home or private hospital have been used up the operation list must be suspended until they have been replaced.

5. The nursing homes or private hospitals should have suitable blood refrigerators solely reserved for blood storage. The supplies of blood should be supervised by a haematologist and made available for recycling if possible.

CHAPTER 7

Genital Tract Sepsis

Summary

There were six Direct deaths due to genital tract sepsis and three others in which sepsis played a major role, but are counted under spontaneous abortion (two deaths) and ectopic pregnancy (one death). The causative organisms were identified as *Group A beta-haemolytic streptococci* in four deaths and *E. coli* in two.

Genital tract sepsis

There were six deaths due to infection of the genital tract and three other Direct deaths in which sepsis occurred — two following spontaneous abortion and one following ectopic pregnancy. All three are discussed in Chapter 6.

The causative organism was identified in all six instances. It was *group A haemolytic streptococcus* in four cases and *E. coli* in two. An *E. coli* peritonitis was present in one of the three deaths discussed in Chapter 6 in a woman with a missed abortion.

Of the six counted deaths two women died undelivered, two had normal deliveries and two were delivered by Caesarean section. The deaths of the nine women in which sepsis occurred have been classified as follows:–

Sepsis after unspecified abortion	ICD 637.0	1
Sepsis and damage to pelvic organs with missed abortion	ICD 639.2	1
Sepsis after ectopic abdominal pregnancy	ICD 639.0	1
Sepsis in pregnancy	ICD 646.6 and 647.8	2
Sepsis after surgical procedures	ICD 670.0	2
Puerperal sepsis	ICD 670.0	2

Table 7.1 shows the continuing low number of deaths from sepsis from all causes.

Streptococcal infections

The diagnosis was not made before death in any of the four women, but all had blood cultures taken before they died. The interval from the first symptoms of infection to death was short. Brief details of these cases are as follows:

Table 7.1 *Maternal deaths from genital tract sepsis including abortion and ectopic pregnancy with rates per million maternities, England and Wales 1970–87, compared with United Kingdom 1985–87.*

	Triennium	Sepsis after abortion	Sepsis after ectopic pregnancy	Puerperal sepsis	Sepsis after surgical procedures	Sepsis before or during labour	Total	Rate per million maternities
England	1970–72	36	—	13	16	1	66	28.7
& Wales	1973–75	6	—	8	11	—	25	13.0
	1976–78	7	—	6	9	—	22	12.6
	1979–81	7	—	2	4	2	15	7.8
	1982–84	3	—	—	1	1	5	2.7
	1985–87	2	1	2	2	2	9	4.5
United Kingdom	1985–87	2	1	2	2	2	9	4.0

A primigravida had an uneventful pregnancy being seen by the consultant or senior registrar at each hospital visit. She was admitted in labour at term, with a history of diarrhoea and vomiting in the preceding 24 hours. She had a temperature of 38°C throughout a short labour in the early hours of the morning. After delivery she was barrier nursed. At a change of duty round a senior house officer (SHO) noted that the women was very ill and hyperventilating, and suspected that she might have toxic shock due to infection. Whilst the SHO left the room to organise equipment to take blood samples the woman had a cardio-respiratory arrest for which immediate resuscitation was carried out. The woman was moved to theatre with a view to carrying out an embolectomy as the diagnosis was considered to be pulmonary embolism. During a cardiorespiratory support by-pass it was noted that the woman was extremely toxic and a laparotomy was performed. There was 200 ml of blood-stained purulent free fluid in the abdomen. The uterus was dark in colour with a black patch on its anterior surface. The small bowel also had an area of scattered black patches present. Despite active resuscitative measures the woman died 36 hours after delivery. A detailed autopsy revealed haemolytic streptococci in the maternal blood, high vaginal swab, urine, peritoneal fluid and gut. The same organism was isolated from the baby's nose, throat, umbilicus and stool. The infant was given antibiotics and did not develop any sign of infection.

A parous woman was admitted in the second stage of labour at term with a history of pyrexia for 1–2 days. A stillborn infant was delivered soon after admission and the third stage was uneventful. There was mild post-delivery pyrexia and the woman felt dizzy, with backache and lower abdominal pain. Shortly afterwards bleeding started due to a coagulation defect which could not be corrected. Despite hysterectomy the woman died from profound septicaemia. *Beta-haemolytic streptococci* were cultured from the maternal blood and uterus taken during life and also from the stillborn baby.

A parous woman was admitted after an uncomplicated pregnancy at term with a history of spontaneous rupture of membranes. Caesarean section was carried out because of slow progress in labour and irregularity of the fetal heart. The day after delivery the mother was transferred to a medical ward because of breathlessness. There was erythema around the abdominal wound and she was treated as a case of septicaemia, with intravenous antibiotics. The following day she had a sudden cardiac arrest with, despite successful resuscitation, a severe degree of cerebral anoxia, and she died three weeks later. *Beta-haemolytic streptococci* were grown from both the maternal blood and from the Caesarean section wound.

A parous woman had an uneventful pregnancy until admitted at 33–34 weeks in a collapsed, shocked and cyanosed state. There was a two-day history of sore throat, vomiting and diarrhoea. Fetal movements had not been felt for 24 hours. Despite intensive resuscitation procedures she had a cardiac arrest and died. The disease process was associated with intravascular haemolysis. Cultures from the placenta and large bowel were positive for *Group A beta-haemolytic streptococcus*.

All four cases indicate the rapid progression of streptococcal septicaemia and the association of disseminated intravascular coagulopathy (DIC).

Infections due to *E. coli*

A parous woman had a Caesarean section because of failure to progress in labour after 12 hours. No details were provided of the length of time the membranes were ruptured, the dilatation of the cervix or whether there was a pyrexia. The woman was transferred to the intensive care unit shortly after delivery, but no reason was given. Her condition gradually deteriorated due to progressive sepsis and DIC developed. A laparotomy was carried out on the third day of the puerperium and an obviously infected uterus was removed but the woman died later that day. Cultures from the uterus at the time of the hysterectomy and from multiple sites of the baby grew *E. coli*. The details given by the consultant obstetrician on the MCW97 form were minimal and the report was regarded as substandard.

A young, parous woman had premature rupture of the membranes three days prior to admission. She was admitted at 24 weeks' gestation with abdominal pain, pyrexia and tachycardia associated with a severe herpes simplex infection of the cervix, vagina and vulva. The uterus was tender and there was ulceration of the lower genital tract. Intravenous antibiotics were commenced immediately followed by acyclovir. Contractions commenced four hours later, but her condition deteriorated and over the next eight hours she had a rigor, hyperpyrexia, cyanosis and finally cardiac arrest. She died undelivered the day after admission of gram negative septicaemia with early intravascular coagulation.

The autopsy both histologically and microbiologically confirmed the presence of an *E. coli* septicaemia.

Substandard care

Whenever sepsis is suspected it is essential that blood cultures are taken and the results of the final reports made available to the Assessors. Failure by all those involved to provide details of the case for the Confidential Enquiries for those women who actually or possibly die from genital tract sepsis must be regarded as substandard.

Discussion

The possibility of infection and sepsis tends to be forgotten in an era of widely available antibiotics and use of prophylactic antibiotic therapy. Genital sepsis is a cause of maternal morbidity and mortality which needs to be constantly remembered since it is often insidious in its onset and can be rapidly fulminating in its outcome.

The cases of genital tract infection resulting in death in this triennium indicate the considerable risk. *Group A haemolytic streptococci* have been responsible for epidemics of puerperal infection through the ages. The severity of the infection is dependent upon both the virulence of the organism and the resistance of the patient. The pathological feature of a Group A beta haemolytic streptococcal genital infection is that spread outside the uterus is rapid. The immune response to the infection is poor so that septicaemia occurs early with little evidence of local reaction at the placental site, the uterus and pelvic peritoneum. In fulminating puerperal infections the temperature may not be raised despite collapse of the patient.

Early accurate bacteriological diagnosis is vital as is treatment with the appropriate antibiotics. The initial treatment must be broad-spectrum and include cover for anaerobes and streptococci, for example amoxycillin-clavulanate and metronidazole plus an aminoglycoside such as gentamicin or a third generation cephalosporin. Obviously the advice of a micro-biologist should be obtained as soon as practicable. Once the organisms are identified more appropriate antibiotics can be given if there is little or no response to the initial antibiotics prescribed.

CHAPTER 8

Genital Tract Trauma

Summary

This chapter includes deaths from uterine rupture and also those deaths dealt with under the heading of 'Other Obstetric Trauma' in the chapter on haemorrhage in previous reports for England and Wales. Under this heading are included all maternal deaths considered to be the direct result of trauma to the genital tract, including vaginal, cervical and uterine tears whether spontaneous or through a previous uterine scar. There were six such cases in this triennium which can be compared with three uterine ruptures and two other obstetric trauma in England and Wales in 1982/84. In all these six cases the uterus was significantly involved although in four the trauma was primarily cervical. Care was considered to be substandard in all six.

Genital tract trauma

Of the six Direct deaths due to genital tract trauma two were due to uterine rupture occurring spontaneously during normal labour. Four were caused by cervical lacerations, one due to oxytocic over-stimulation and three to instrumental extraction (two ventouse, one forceps) through a scarred or incompletely dilated cervix (Table 8.1). All involved the uterus but as in the previous two triennia for England and Wales there were no ruptured Caesarean section scars leading to maternal death.

Table 8.1 *Trends in mortality from ruptured uterus 1970–87.*

		Spontaneous	Induced			Total	Rate per million maternities
			Oxytocic	Instrumental	Manipulative		
England	1970–72	3	6	2	—	11	4.8
& Wales	1973–75	5	3	2	1	11	5.7
	1976–78	5	4	4	1	14	8.0
	1979–81	1	3	—	—	4	7.3
	1982–84	—	2	—	1*	3	1.6
	1985–87	2	—	3	—	5	2.5
United Kingdom	1985–87	2	1	3	—	6	2.7

* One case — doubtful classification because of insufficient information

In addition to these six Direct deaths there was a spontaneous rupture of the uterus associated with sepsis and a missed abortion which is counted and discussed in Chapter 6.

Spontaneous uterine rupture

This occurred on two occasions. Care was considered to be substandard in both.

The first involved a multipara, who having delivered herself rapidly of a large infant sustained a profuse postpartum haemorrhage estimated at 4.5 litres in 10 minutes. Resuscitation was begun and vaginal examination under anaesthesia by the registrar failed to diagnose what at autopsy was found to be 'an extensive ragged rupture of the lower uterine segment'. The haemorrhage was not controlled by the administration of 13.5 litres of IV fluid including 4 litres of blood, and 5.5 litres of blood products. Disseminated intravascular coagulation (DIC) was diagnosed. The consultant obstetrician was informed and first saw the patient when the registrar had already started an exploratory laparotomy. The patient died on the operating table soon afterwards. Autopsy confirmed uterine rupture and DIC due to amniotic fluid embolism.

The second spontaneous rupture occurred in a multipara. She was treated in hospital for recurring vaginal bleeding during the second trimester. On her third admission her haemoglobin concentration was 7.7g/dl and she was given 1.5 litres of blood. Vaginal bleeding persisted and a few days after admission she suddenly became shocked. The senior house officer began resuscitation with IV saline, followed two hours later by blood, but the patient's condition deteriorated and she died undelivered. Only then were the registrar and the consultant informed. Autopsy showed that the primary cause of death was massive retroperitoneal haemorrhage extending upwards to surround the spleen and left kidney, secondary to uterine rupture for which no definite cause was apparent. There was also evidence in the lungs of amniotic fluid embolism.

Traumatic uterine rupture

This occurred on four occasions; all had primary cervical lacerations. Oxytocin had been administered during the first stage in all four and its use played a significant part in the uterine rupture in one and may have been a factor in another.

A woman had had sustained extensive tearing of the upper vagina and cervix causing postpartum haemorrhage in a previous pregnancy. In this pregnancy her haemoglobin concentration gradually fell after the 30th week and at the 36th week was 9.9g/dl; haematinics were not given. She was admitted in labour at term when amniotomy was performed followed by *Syntocinon* infusion. She was delivered spontaneously after a short labour but following a normal third stage haemorrhage occurred and persisted. She collapsed about an hour after delivery. The registrar diagnosed a cervical laceration and inserted one suture in the cervix which failed to control the bleeding. Three hours after the haemorrhage had begun the consultant was called and a laparotomy confirmed a cervical tear extending into the lower uterine segment associated with a broad ligament haematoma. Hysterectomy failed to control the bleeding although there was no apparent clotting defect. Despite attempts at resuscitation by the anaesthetic registrar she died within 12 hours of delivery. Autopsy showed no evidence of DIC or amniotic embolism.

An obese young woman, who had previously been delivered by Caesarean section for fetal distress, refused antenatal care at hospital but was seen regularly by a midwife at home. At term she was admitted in labour; because progress was slow in the first seven hours the locum registrar suggested that Caesarean section should be performed if there was no advance. Three hours later however, the cervix having failed to dilate beyond four cm, it was decided to augment labour with *Syntocinon*. This caused strong painful contractions and because of this was discontinued after one hour. When the caput was visible a forceps delivery was performed for fetal bradycardia. Immediately after suture of the episiotomy the patient collapsed. The consultant obstetrician was called and diagnosed rupture of the uterus for which he performed a laparotomy. It was then evident that although the scar of the previous Caesarean section was intact the cervix had torn up into the lower uterine segment and down into the vagina to join the upper end of the episiotomy. Hysterectomy was performed but haemostasis was unsatisfactory and despite vigorous and expert resuscitative measures under the supervision of a consultant anaesthetist the patient's heart stopped on two occasions. She then showed evidence of brainstem death and died two days after delivery. Autopsy confirmed extensive tearing of the vagina, cervix and lower uterine segment and indicated that the upper 6cm of the vaginal tear was 'largely open'. There was no evidence of clotting defect.

In the other two cases of cervical laceration where oxytocin was used in labour this did not have any causative effect on the lesion. In both of these the cervical tear was directly due to the use of the ventouse through an incompletely dilated cervix.

A parous woman with a history of eclampsia and postpartum haemorrhage was admitted at term with oedema and hypertension. Labour began spontaneously two days later. The fetal head remained high and amniotomy was performed and IV *Syntocinon* administered. Two hours later the fetal heart slowed to under 90/min. The patient was therefore delivered by ventouse through an 8cm dilated cervix. Immediately thereafter there was a gush of blood from the vagina and the patient collapsed. A diagnosis of intrapartum placental abruption was made and resuscitation with IV fluids and blood commenced. Initial improvement was not maintained and shock deepened despite expert resuscitative measures. Five hours after delivery she was seen by the consultant obstetrician who, on vaginal examination, diagnosed a cervical tear extending into the lower uterine segment. Abdominal hysterectomy was performed but the patient failed to respond to resuscitation in the Intensive Care Unit (ICU) and died eight hours later. Autopsy was not performed.

A young woman was admitted to hospital before term with spontaneous rupture of the membranes. Labour ensued and was augmented with *Syntocinon*; after 11 hours, she was delivered by a senior house officer

(SHO) with the ventouse because of an irregular fetal heart. Despite IV ergometrine there was persistent postpartum vaginal bleeding. There was a delay in the request for blood and a further delay before it became available approximately six hours after delivery. Examination under anaesthesia by the SHO disclosed a large volume of blood clot in the vagina coming from a 'ragged' cervix; the uterus was empty and well contracted. Two catgut sutures were inserted in the cervix. An hour and a half later the patient, who remained hypovolaemic and had not yet recovered from the anaesthetic administered by a registrar, developed cardiac arrest which was successfully treated by the cardiac arrest team. Central venous pressure monitoring had not been used. Heavy vaginal bleeding occurred and the consultant obstetrician was informed. Control of the bleeding was achieved with difficulty and resuscitative measures, including 13 units of blood, succeeded in stabilising the patient's condition. She was then transferred to the ICU where eight hours after the cardiac arrest she developed convulsions. She died about a week later. Autopsy showed extensive haemorrhage in the basal ganglia and evidence of DIC. The cervix uteri was severely damaged and showed acute necrosis and haemorrhage throughout, and a tear of the left posterior lip which, although sutured, had continued to bleed.

Pathology

Five of these six cases came to autopsy. In four there was a full anatomical description, with appropriate histology; in two of these, where a hysterectomy had been carried out prior to death, a full report on the separate surgical specimen was included.

In the fifth case, the autopsy report was no more than adequate. There was no description of the histological findings, although tissue for histology was apparently taken, nor of the previously resected uterus.

In the sixth case, it was reported that autopsy permission was refused, but this early post-operative maternal death should certainly have fallen within the Coroner's jurisdiction.

Substandard care

This was considered to be a factor in all the deaths from genital tract trauma and was most significant in the traumatic ruptures. Significant anaemia was left untreated in three patients despite regular antenatal care. The most important lapses in intrapartum management were the inexperience of the doctors in charge resulting in poor obstetric diagnosis and operative technique; more expert assistance was sometimes unsought or delayed. Misuse of *Syntocinon* was responsible for one uterine rupture and may have played a part in another. Three ruptures were associated with instrumental deliveries, one with forceps and two with the ventouse. Compatible blood was sometimes only available after considerable delay. Resuscitation was deficient in two cases managed solely by junior staff.

Discussion

It is of paramount importance that patients known to be seriously at risk of uterine rupture should only be admitted to fully staffed and equipped hospitals where experienced obstetric and anaesthetic assistance and intensive care are always readily available.

Serious trauma of the genital tract and failure to recognise and treat it efficiently in time to save life were usually the result of the inexperience of the doctor in charge. especially important was failure to engage more expert assistance early, whether obstetric for accurate diagnosis and control of haemorrhage, or anaesthetic for efficient resuscitation. Anaemia, especially in high risk patients, the abuse of *Syntocinon* and the extraction of the fetus with forceps or ventouse through a cervix scarred or not fully dilated also played a significant part in these tragic cases. To prevent them in future triennia requires nothing more complicated than vigilance and appropriate clinical and administrative endeavour.

CHAPTER 9

Deaths associated with anaesthesia

Summary

There were six deaths directly attributable to anaesthesia during this triennium. There were also two Late deaths which were directly due to anaesthesia. Four of the six deaths, and the two Late deaths, were due to problems associated with tracheal intubation. The other two deaths were respectively due to the inhalation of gastric contents at induction of anaesthesia and to cardiovascular collapse resulting from an epidural anaesthetic in a patient with severe congenital heart disease.

Anaesthesia was considered to have contributed to death in a further 16 women. Five of the deaths were associated with cardiac disease, four with haemorrhage, three with hypertensive disorders of pregnancy, and the remaining four with miscellaneous conditions. In five of these 16 patients there was a failure in the provision of adequate postoperative care.

Although there has been a reduction in the number of deaths directly attributable to anaesthesia since the last report for England and Wales, there is still a high incidence of tracheal tube problems. A failure of organisation and postoperative care was frequently identified, and in many situations monitoring was inadequate. There is a need to concentrate resources in units where consultant cover can be provided continuously, and to identify patients at risk before anaesthesia is induced.

Deaths associated with anaesthesia

In the 1985–87 triennium there were 22 deaths associated with anaesthesia, six of the deaths being directly attributable to anaesthesia and 16 in which anaesthesia was considered to have contributed to death. In addition, there were two deaths directly due to anaesthesia which are classified as Late Deaths (Chapter 15). Deaths have again been classified as ICD 668 ('Complications of the administration of anaesthetic or other sedation in labour and delivery'). The figures for this triennium include those for Scotland and Northern Ireland for the first time but it is still not possible to determine the true mortality rate since the total number of anaesthetics given for obstetric conditions is unknown. However, it is believed that since the total number of anaesthetics given for abortion and operative delivery has increased, the figures shown in Table 9.1 represent a real decrease in deaths directly attributable to anaesthesia.

Table 9.1 *Deaths, associated with anaesthesia, estimated rate per million pregnancies and percentage of Direct maternal deaths England and Wales 1970–87, compared with United Kingdom 1985–87.*

		Number of deaths directly associated with anaesthesia	Rate per million pregnancies	% of Direct maternal deaths
England & Wales	1970–72	37	12.8	10.8
	1973–75	27	10.5	11.9
	1976–78	27	12.1	12.4
	1979–81	22	8.7	12.4
	1982–84	18	7.2	13.0
	1985–87	5	1.9	4.4
United Kingdom	1985–87	6	N/A	4.3

Deaths directly due to anaesthesia

Table 9.2 summarises the causes of death in the eight patients including the two Late deaths in whom anaesthesia was considered to be the main cause of death. Six of these were associated directly or indirectly with problems arising from tracheal intubation. Two of the patients were of short stature and four were described as obese.

Table 9.2 *Direct deaths attributable to anaesthesia: procedures for which anaesthesia was given*

Operation	Indication	Cause of death	Number of deaths
Elective Caesarean section	Cephalopelvic disproportion	Misplaced tracheal tube	1)
	Aortic incompetence	Epidural/cardiovascular collapse	1)) 2
Emergency planned Caesarean section	Fetal distress	Misplaced tracheal tube	1)
	Failure to progress, breech	Misplaced tracheal tube	1)) 2
Emergency unplanned Caesarean section	Previous Caesarean section. ?Ruptured uterus	Aspiration of gastric contents	1
Manual removal of placenta	Retained placenta	Kinked tracheal tube	1
Late deaths			
Elective Caesarean section	Cephalopelvic dysproportion	Misplaced tracheal tube, respiratory arrest secondary to complication of epidural anaesthesia.	1
Emergency Caesarean section	Fetal distress	Misplaced tracheal tube	1

Difficulty with tracheal intubation

The first woman, who had undergone a Caesarean section previously, was scheduled for an elective Caesarean section for cephalopelvic disproportion. She was offered an epidural but chose a general anaesthetic.

She was appropriately prepared and general anaesthesia was administered using a standard technique with muscle relaxants. Although the intubation was difficult there was a failure to accept that the tube was in the oesophagus until anoxia caused cardiac arrest and the patient died.

The second woman was obese and had been given ineffective epidural anaesthesia in a previous pregnancy. She was in labour with a breech presentation and a trial of vaginal delivery under epidural anaesthesia was planned. The epidural gave good pain relief during labour and she progressed to full dilatation of the cervix. There was no progress in the second stage and the obstetrician considered that Caesarean section was indicated. The epidural had not been topped up for two hours and so a total of 30ml of 0.5% bupivacaine was given in divided doses over 30 minutes. However, this did not provide adequate anaesthesia for Caesarean section. General anaesthesia was induced, the vocal cords were not visualised at laryngoscopy but intubation of the trachea was thought to have been achieved using a gum elastic bougie as an introducer. It was stated that the registrar anaesthetist had neither a skilled nurse nor an operating department assistant in attendance. Alcuronium 20mg was given on return of muscle power but there was no record of the return of spontaneous respiration or of movements of the reservoir bag. Hypoxia developed, the tube was removed and the patient was manually ventilated with a mask. However, cardiac arrest occurred and during the resuscitation the consultant obstetrician arrived and delivered the baby by breech extraction. Death occurred two days later in the intensive care unit (ICU) as a result of the hypoxic episode.

The third woman, described as grossly obese, had had previous normal deliveries. She was hypertensive, oedematous and had proteinuria. Labour was induced at term in the hope that vaginal delivery would be achieved. She received intravenous hydralazine to control her blood pressure during labour. She made slow progress and after 19 hours of labour, when the cervix was 8cm dilated, signs of fetal distress developed and Caesarean section was considered necessary. General anaesthesia was induced by an experienced anaesthetist, but although intubation was difficult the tube was thought to be in the trachea. Breath sounds were audible. Cardiac arrest occurred during the Caesarean section in a markedly cyanosed patient. She could not be resuscitated. Tracheostomy was attempted but not achieved by the consultant obstetrician. All the staff were convinced that the tube was in the trachea though the trachea was never opened. Again, suxamethonium had been followed by a non-depolarising muscle relaxant without observing the return of spontaneous respiration.

The fourth woman was admitted in labour with a concealed pregnancy. The diastolic pressure was 110m Hg and no fetal heartbeat was heard. She received hydralazine intravenously and was delivered of a still-born infant. The placenta was retained. General anaesthesia, which included thiopentone, suxamethonium, alfentanil and vecuronium, was administered by a junior anaesthetist. The patient failed to breathe postoperatively and suxamethonium sensitivity was suspected. She was transferred to a high-dependency unit for mechanical ventilation but 15 minutes later high inflation pressures were recorded and it was considered that her tracheal tube had become obstructed, probably by kinking. Hypoventilation resulted in irreversible brain damage before the tube was inspected and changed. She did not regain consciousness and died a week later. Autopsy revealed pulmonary hypertensive disease but death was considered to be due to hypoxia secondary to an obstructed endotracheal tube.

Late deaths

The remaining two Direct deaths, which were also associated with tracheal tube problems, are classified as Late deaths and included in Chapter 15.

One woman received an urgent general anaesthetic for Caesarean section because of fetal distress in labour. The anaesthetist was a locum registrar and again there was failure to accept that the tracheal tube was in the oesophagus. By the time experienced anaesthetic assistance had arrived, hypoxia had caused irreversible brain damage. The patient survived for many months following the Caesarean section without regaining consciousness.

The second woman died more than six months after an elective Caesarean section for cephalopelvic disproportion. She had previously had a Caesarean section for cephalopelvic disproportion under general anaesthesia, at which time it had been recorded that tracheal intubation could not be achieved by direct laryngoscopy and that she had required a blind nasal intubation under inhalational anaesthesia. She was not seen by an anaesthetist until the morning of the planned Caesarean section and again a consultant anaesthetist was not able to intubate her trachea under direct vision. She was awakened and an epidural anaesthetic was given by an experienced junior anaesthetist who was not directly supervised. A test dose of 2ml 1% lignocaine was negative and 8ml 0.5% bupivacaine was then administered through the epidural catheter. The blood pressure dropped acutely and was maintained with intravenous ephedrine and fluid. There was increasing difficulty in breathing and spontaneous respiration eventually ceased. Attempts at tracheal intubation were initially unsuccessful and the tube was then misplaced in the oesophagus. The error was not recognised for some time but eventually the tube was removed and adequate ventilation achieved with a mask. Senior anaesthetic assistance had been summoned and a consultant anaesthetist eventually achieved tracheal intubation. A stillborn infant was delivered by Caesarean section but the patient suffered severe permanent neurological impairment which resulted in her eventual death.

Comment

Five of the six deaths due to tracheal tube problems were associated with unrecognised misplacement of the tracheal tube. It is well recognised that there are a number of anatomical factors which may make tracheal intubation difficult. However, there are additional factors which increase the difficulties in obstetric anaesthesia. The intubation often has to be performed at short notice, there is frequently a lack of skilled assistance, the larynx and soft tissues may be swollen by fluid retention and the position of the larynx may be changed by the incorrect application of cricoid pressure. It is also not generally appreciated that the larynx may close and the arytenoid cartilages may move anteriorly if laryngoscopy is performed when the patient is inadequately anaesthetised, even though a normal dose of muscle relaxant has been given. It is, therefore, important to ensure that the patient is adequately anaesthetised, that there is a full range of equipment for dealing with a difficult intubation, and that adequate skilled anaesthetic assistance is provided. Cricoid pressures requires the use of two hands, one hand pressing the cricoid cartilage whilst the neck is supported and maintained in the intubating position with the other. This demands the sole attention of the attending midwife, who has been trained in the technique, and frees the anaesthetic assistant to provide equipment which may be urgently required in the event of a difficult intubation. A failed intubation drill should be agreed and practised by all those involved in obstetric anaesthesia.

The extra anaesthetic apparatus required for a difficult intubation includes:

1. a laryngoscope with a blade in line with the axis of the handle (polio blade);

2. long introducers (gum-elastic, rubber or plastic coated malleable wire);

3. laryngeal masks;

4. large bore oro-gastric tubes;

5. a laryngotomy kit.

The use of the fibre-optic laryngoscope as an introducer should be restricted to those who have practised the technique. It should be noted that a laryngeal mask does not protect the airway against regurgitated stomach contents and its use in obstetric patients must be accompanied by the continued application of cricoid pressure[1]. If an anaesthetist fails to intubate the trachea and cannot maintain a satisfactory airway with continued cricoid pressure priority should be given to the mother's safety and she should be allowed to recover consciousness.

Inhalation of stomach contents

In this triennium only one woman died directly as a result of aspiration of stomach contents into the lungs in association with anaesthesia.

A woman, who had undergone a Caesarean section previously, went into spontaneous labour and received opioid analgesia during labour. Her labour failed to progress and rupture of the uterus was considered a possibility. She received a general anaesthetic for an emergency Caesarean section. She had received oral ranitidine during labour and subsequently received intravenous ranitidine and oral sodium citrate just prior to induction of anaesthesia. Regurgitation occurred at the time of induction and aspiration pneumonitis ensued despite an accepted method of antacid prophylaxis. A skilled anaesthetic assistant was present and cricoid pressure was applied though it is not possible to ascertain whether the manoeuvre was properly performed.

Cardiac disease

One death was considered to be directly attributable to the anaesthetic in a woman with congenital heart disease.

A primigravida had aortic valve incompetence complicated by heart failure and pre-eclampsia. She had proteinuria, dependent oedema and dyspnoea. She was treated with methyldopa and frusemide orally. It was decided to deliver her at 32 weeks gestation by Caesarean section under epidural anaesthesia because of increasing cardiac failure. Epidural anaesthesia was induced after an intravenous preload of 1 litre of Hartmann's solution. A test dose of 2ml of 0.5% bupivacaine was followed by a single bolus infection of 18ml 0.5% bupivacaine through an epidural catheter at the L3/4 interspace. A further 6ml 0.5% bupivacaine was then given because of deficient sacral root blockade but profound cardiovascular collapse occurred. The upper sensory level of block was considered to be T4. Further intravenous fluid and 15mg intravenous ephedrine were administered with minimal effect. Ventricular fibrillation ensued, resuscitation was unsuccessful and she died within two hours of the initial collapse. Autopsy findings confirmed the clinical diagnosis of aortic incompetence with left ventricular hypertrophy.

Comment

The management of patients with cardiac disease should be the joint responsibility of the cardiologist and obstetrician but the consultant anaesthetist should be involved at an early stage of pregnancy in case anaesthesia is required during pregnancy. The choice of anaesthetic in patients who are either in, or on the verge of, cardiac failure, is controversial. Although it has been argued that patients with aortic incompetence may benefit from a reduction in peripheral vascular resistance it is important to maintain a normal diastolic pressure so that coronary blood flow to the subendocardium of the hypertrophied left ventricle is not reduced. Perioperative measurements of venous and arterial pressure are essential whilst monitoring of the pulmonary artery wedge pressure during the gradual establishment of neural blockade, by fractionating the dose of local anaesthetic, might have helped in this particular case. Careful monitoring of vascular pressures would have allowed accurate titration of intravenous fluids, vasoconstrictor or inotropic agents and avoided sudden decompensation of the circulation. General anaesthesia might have prevented the profound hypotension which resulted from sudden sympathetic blockade but again, invasive monitoring would have been appropriate.

Deaths to which anaesthesia contributed

These are summarised in Table 9.3 and are also discussed in the relevant chapters of the report.

Table 9.3 *Main cause of death where anaesthetic factors contributed to death (excluding deaths directly due to anaesthesia)*

Cause of death	Number	Chapter
Hypertensive disorders	3	Chapter 2
Haemorrhage	2	Chapter 3
Early pregnancy deaths	1	Chapter 6
Genital tract trauma	2	Chapter 8
Other Direct deaths	2	Chapter 10*
Cardiac deaths	5	Chapter 11
Indirect: phaeochromocytoma	1	Chapter 12
Total	16	

* Includes unexplained death following legal abortion.

Hypertensive disorders of pregnancy

There were three women with pre-eclampsia in whom the management of the anaesthetic or sedation was thought to have contributed to death. Two of these deaths were secondary to events which occurred in the postoperative period and are considered in that section. One death, which occurred as a result of sedation during labour, is considered here.

A woman was admitted with severe pre-eclampsia at 26 weeks gestation. She received intravenous hydralazine and chlormethiazole to control the blood pressure and provide sedation. Labour was induced and 100 mg pethidine injected intramuscularly to provide analgesia. About an hour later she was deeply sedated and suffered an episode of airway obstruction. The duration of this episode was not defined although the anaesthetist was in attendance. There did not appear to have been any further problems with the airway although the patient remained heavily sedated. She had a normal delivery but postpartum was unconscious, oedematous and had a poor urine output. She was, therefore, transferred to an ICU in another hospital. She died of progressive respiratory failure secondary to the adult respiratory distress syndrome (ARDS) in the third postpartum week. The cause of the ARDS was not clear but may have been due to unobserved aspiration of stomach contents in the unconscious patient.

Comment

The administration of a potent sedative such as chlormethiazole in combination with an opioid results in sedation progressing to a state of general anaesthesia. This level of sedation carries a high risk of aspiration or airway obstruction which can only be minimised by the provision of continuous skilled nursing care under the supervision of the anaesthetist.

Haemorrhage and genital tract trauma

Substandard anaesthetic care was considered to have contributed to the deaths of four women who died from haemorrhage. Two of these cases are counted in Chapter 3 and two in Chapter 8. One death from postpartum haemorrhage and two from genital tract trauma are considered here and the fourth death is discussed in the section on postoperative care.

One woman who died of a secondary postpartum haemorrhage during evacuation of the uterus, refused blood or blood products because of her religious belief. Though this was the primary reason for death, failure to administer adequate volumes of crystalloid or colloid and failure to monitor the central venous pressure contributed.

Two women died from postpartum haemorrhage secondary to cervical tears. In the first case no blood had been crossmatched though she was known to be anaemic and had a history of severe genital tract trauma at a previous delivery. Advice was sought from a consultant anaesthetist but the registrar was left to carry out the anaesthesia and resuscitation alone. Monitoring and transfusion were inadequate and she died whilst being taken back to theatre for ligation of the internal iliac arteries. In the second woman blood loss was again underestimated and replacement was inadequate before and during the general anaesthetic. Monitoring was inadequate and the dose of anaesthetic agent may have been excessive for a patient in hypovolaemic shock.

Comment

Fluid replacement in haemorrhage should not be delayed until a fall in arterial pressure occurs, for this is a relatively late sign of hypovolaemia and indicates that compensatory mechanisms have been exhausted. When excessive bleeding occurs a central venous line should be inserted immediately and direct monitoring of arterial pressure instituted if possible. At least two large bore venous cannulae should be inserted, the blood bank alerted to provide blood, fresh frozen plasma and platelets, and extra assistance sought (Annex, Chapter 3).

Cardiac disease

There were five deaths in patients with cardiac disease in which anaesthesia was considered to have contributed to death. Three of these occurred in women with congenital heart disease and two were associated with ischaemic heart disease. Two patients, one with primary pulmonary hypertension and one with residual pulmonary hypertension after open heart surgery, died during labour under epidural anaesthesia.

The first woman suffered a cardiac arrest during manual removal of the placenta. This was probably precipitated by an acute increase in pulmonary artery pressure secondary to the sudden increase in blood volume produced by contraction of the uterus.

The second woman had a cardiac arrest following an epidural top-up of 5ml of 0.25% bupivacaine. This was probably associated with a reduction in right ventricular filling pressure produced by the sympathetic blockade.

Comment

Patients with pulmonary hypertension have large changes in pulmonary artery pressure when cardiac output is changed or pulmonary vasoactive drugs are given. It is, therefore, essential to maintain constant right ventricular filling pressures with central venous pressure monitoring and consideration should be given to the insertion of a flow-directed (Swan-Ganz) pulmonary artery catheter. In such patients oxytocic drugs should *not* be given *except* in the presence of severe haemorrhage due to uterine atony, and then only with extreme caution.

A third woman with congenital heart disease had previously undergone aortic valve replacement. During the pregnancy she developed infective endocarditis on the prosthetic tissue valve causing incompetence and left ventricular failure. It was planned that a Caesarean section should be performed at 33 weeks gestation and that this should be followed by an early postpartum valve replacement. An experienced anaesthetist gave her a general anaesthetic for the Caesarean section which was completed uneventfully. Despite this careful management, she suddenly collapsed and died during recovery. Autopsy revealed that the aortic prosthesis had become detached and had wedged in the aortic bifurcation.

Comment

It is apparent with hindsight that complicated cases of this type should be delivered in a unit where all the facilities are available for immediate cardiac surgery.

One of the two patients with ischaemic heart disease is discussed in the section on postoperative problems.

The other was an elderly multiparous woman with gestational diabetes and a previous history of angina who underwent Caesarean section for fetal distress. Blood pressure during labour had been elevated, with a diastolic of 110mm Hg, but had not been recorded before induction of anaesthesia. An electrocardiogram (ECG) had not been ordered in the antenatal period or early labour, in spite of the history. Following induction of anaesthesia the woman became acutely hypotensive with evidence of myocardial ischaemia on the ECG monitor. She suffered a cardiac arrest following delivery of the baby. Autopsy confirmed a massive myocardial infarction with severe coronary artery disease.

Comment

The woman's age and history should have alerted the obstetric and anaesthetic staff to the increased risk and a pre-delivery ECG would have been valuable. The decrease in blood pressure may have been secondary to aortocaval obstruction, vasodilatation or myocardial depression secondary to general anesthesia but it did not appear to be due to blood loss. A rapid sequence induction may be hazardous in patients with significant myocardial ischaemia and careful monitoring of arterial blood pressure and its maintenance by physical or pharmacological means is essential.

Other deaths

Four deaths in this group are also counted in other chapters. One was an 'Early pregnancy death', two were 'Other Direct deaths' and one was an Indirect death. Three of these patients are considered here and one Other Direct death is considered later under failure of post-operative care.

The early pregnancy death occurred in a woman with sickle-cell trait who died following laparotomy for a ruptured tubal pregnancy. She was anaemic before surgery with a haemoglobin concentration of 4.6g/dl and had sustained a large blood loss. She suffered an episode of pulmonary oedema during anaesthesia which was presumed to be due to circulatory overload from overtransfusion in the absence of central venous pressure monitoring. A central venous line was eventually inserted but death was considered to be due to pulmonary oedema.

Comment

The replacement of major blood loss with blood, blood products or plasma substitutes requires early measurement and control of the central venous pressure to prevent circulatory overload during transfusion, particularly in the presence of anaemia.

A parous woman had a twin pregnancy and had declined epidural anaesthesia. The first child was delivered uneventfully as an assisted breech but the second child remained high. It was decided to perform a Caesarean section for delivery of the second twin and the anaesthetist, who was not present for the twin delivery, had to be called. A junior obstetrician administered a large dose of salbutamol intravenously and all uterine activity ceased. General anaesthesia was induced but the patient had marked tachycardia. Following delivery of the baby the patient developed severe hypotension and cardiac arrest. There is doubt about the actual cause of death in this case though it is probably that after induction of anaesthesia the cardiac output was compromised due to the large dose of salbutamol, causing tachycardia and arteriolar vasodilatation, possibly combined with aortocaval compression.

Another parous woman was admitted before term in labour but she failed to progress and required Caesarean section. She had received an epidural in labour but this had not been working completely satisfactorily and general anaesthesia was, therefore, induced for the Caesarean section. During the operation the patient exhibited episodes of severe hypertension and supraventricular tachycardia for which she received propranolol intravenously. The blood loss was 1.5 litres and post-operatively there was tachycardia, hypertension and respiratory distress. She continued to deteriorate and suffered cardiac arrest from which she died. A phaeochromocytoma was found at autopsy.

Comment

If the possibility of a phaeochromocytoma had been considered clinically, combined treatment with direct vasodilator or alpha blocking drugs and beta blockade might have controlled her circulation in the postoperative period.

Failure of postoperative care

In five women, failure of care in the postoperative period was considered to have contributed to death. One woman died as a result of acute cardiac failure due to myocardial ischaemia and is counted in Chapter 11. Two died as a result of hypertensive disorders of pregnancy and one as a result of haemorrhage. The fifth woman died during recovery from anaesthesia for an elective termination of pregnancy and is counted as an Other Direct death as there was no satisfactory explanation of the cause of death.

The first woman, who had essential hypertension, developed left ventricular failure secondary to myocardial ischaemia after Caesarean section for placenta praevia. It was apparent that the patient had respiratory problems at the end of the anaesthetic but she was sent to the postnatal ward where she died a few hours later.

A second woman, who had pre-eclampsia, died secondary to an intra-cerebral haemorrhage a few hours after Caesarean section. The post-operative record was incomplete but she was receiving an intravenous infusion of hydralazine for sustained hypertension.

The third woman who also had pre-eclampsia, had an eclamptic fit shortly after Caesarean section. It was clear that the appropriate level of nursing supervision and monitoring of the blood pressure and urine output, which had been requested by the obstetric consultant, had not been provided. She had a further fit and was transferred to an ICU in another hospital. She died two weeks later from progressive respiratory failure secondary to ARDS. It is possible that aspiration of stomach contents occurred at the time of the first fit.

A fourth woman had a postoperative haemorrhage in an inadequately staffed postnatal ward. She had sustained a blood loss of 1–2 litres during surgery. Blood replacement was inadequate and there was a failure to realise that the patient was becoming increasingly shocked due to continued haemorrhage. Death was due to haemorrhage.

The fifth woman, who died after a legal termination of a first trimester pregnancy by suction evacuation of the uterus, had a cardiac arrest within an hour of surgery. A nursing auxiliary was supervising the patient in the recovery area. It is not clear if there was preceding cyanosis or airway obstruction, though the patient had been observed to speak following an uneventful general anaesthetic. There was no record of the immediate postoperative observations and it is not clear if any were carried out. Autopsy revealed severe coronary atheroma but there was no satisfactory explanation of the cause of death.

Comment

These deaths are included in this chapter because anaesthetists now accept a major responsibility for the patient in the immediate postoperative period. This responsibility includes care of the airway, the respiratory and circulatory systems and provision of pain relief. In two of the cases there was a shortage of trained midwives in the postnatal ward. In two other cases there was poor communication between the obstetric and anaesthetic medical staff. This resulted in a failure to provide an appropriate level of care and supervision which was considered to have contributed to the deaths. The fifth death was probably associated with airway obstruction. Nursing and anaesthetic staff often assume that the airway will remain patent when consciousness has returned. However, a number of patients have obstructive episodes with periods of severe desaturation during sleep and the severity of these episodes may be accentuated if the patient is sedated. All heavily sedated or unconscious patients should be nursed in the lateral position and observed continuously. Arterial saturation monitoring by pulse oximetry is strongly recommended. It should be noted however that prolonged periods of airway obstruction may not result in a reduction in arterial saturation if the patient is breathing oxygen. The continuous monitoring of respiration and circulation by trained personnel is therefore mandatory.

Conclusions

The actual reduction in mortality rate directly due to anaesthesia is probably greater than that suggested by the decrease in the number of deaths since the number of anaesthetics for operative procedures continues to rise. The increasing anaesthetic resources devoted to the obstetric service, the increased awareness of the risks of anaesthesia and the increasing use of appropriately supervised regional anesthesia are considered to have contributed to the decline in mortality. However, the occurrence of sixteen deaths in which anaesthesia was considered to be contributory cannot be accepted with complacency. The anaesthetic management in all these cases was considered substandard because there was a failure in clinical care or an administrative failure. The latter includes inappropriate delegation to inexperienced anaesthetists, a lack of adequately trained anaesthetic assistants, and a failure to provide space, staffing and equipment for the implementation of high dependency care. The conclusions reached in this report are similar to those in the 1982–84 report but it should be noted that all the deaths mentioned in this report pre-date the actual publication of that report by at least two years.

The most frequent cause of Direct anaesthetic death in this triennium was failure to intubate the trachea. If this is recognised action can be taken to maintain ventilation by other means. However, if it is not recognised cardiac arrest will occur within a few minutes. In this triennium five women died as a result of misplaced tracheal tubes. These women had been given suxamethonium and a long acting muscle relaxant had then been administered without observing the return of spontaneous respiration. Adequate movements of the reservoir bag help confirm that the tube is in the trachea and eliminate suxamethonium as a cause of postoperative apnoea. Correct placement of the tube should be confirmed immediately after every intubation regardless of whether the tube appears to enter the larynx or not. The anaesthetist should observe the movements of chest and abdomen, listen for the presence of breath sounds in each axilla and confirm that there are no breath sounds over the stomach. The pattern of expansion of the reservoir bag during expiration is also helpful. The oesophageal detector devices also appear to provide a reliable indication of oesophageal intubation[2, 3]. However, the presence of a regular alveolar plateau of carbon dioxide in the expired gas is the only certain method of ensuring that the tube is in the trachea. It is now considered essential that a rapid CO_2 analyser should be provided in every location where anaesthetics are given regularly, so that the position of the tube can be checked immediately after intubation and the adequacy of ventilation monitored throughout the anaesthetic. A pulse oximeter should also be applied during every general anaesthetic though pre-oxygenation may delay the fall in saturation after oesophageal intubation. The other methods of monitoring the anaesthetic apparatus and the patient's condition have been clearly laid down in the Association of Anaesthetists' Recommendations for Monitoring during Anaesthesia and Recovery[4]. These recommendations constitute practical guidelines for minimal monitoring and should form the basis of practice in every obstetric unit where analgesia or anaesthesia is used.

A number of other cases warrant further discussion. The Late Direct death following a complication of epidural anaesthesia was considered to be due to hypoxia resulting from respiratory muscle paralysis caused by profound central neural blockade. Failure to maintain adequate artificial ventilation, because of initial difficulty with tracheal intubation and subsequent incorrect placement of the tube, resulted in gross hypoxia leading to permanent neurological damage. In view of her history, this woman should have been formally referred antenatally for an anaesthetic consultation and her management should not have been left to a junior anaesthetist. The epidural test dose was inadequate to confirm or refute intrathecal placement of the catheter. Total accidental spinal anaesthesia is a recognised complication of epidural anaesthesia and artificial maintenance of the cardiovascular system and respiration should normally not create a problem for an experienced anaesthetist. The additional complication of a misplaced tracheal tube was considered to be the direct cause of death in the patient.

In this report only one woman died as a result of aspiration of stomach contents on induction of anaesthesia as compared with six deaths in the last triennium. However, this decrease could be due to chance. The woman who died had received a commonly used antacid regimen and the failure of this technique to protect against the effects of pulmonary aspiration is disturbing. It may be that pre-operative nasogastric aspiration should still be considered in those patients who have received opioid analgesia during a long labour. It is recommended that all women at risk of losing consciousness should receive antacid prophylaxis. This includes all women who may receive a general anaesthetic and those who may be at risk of eclampsia or loss of consciousness secondary to sedation or to a complication of regional anaesthesia. H_2 receptor blockers should be given early in labour when prophylaxis is considered necessary.

Uncontrolled hypertension at any time during pregnancy is a serious life-threatening condition. The management of labour, operative delivery and postpartum care in the patient with severe pre-eclampsia demands a team approach. It is recognised that it is difficult to identify women who will convulse and this makes management difficult. The anaesthetist is often only consulted when anaesthesia is required but his or her expertise may be useful, particularly when potent sedative drugs are used, or when acute control of arterial hypertension is required during labour. The anaesthetist should also be involved in ensuring that the appropriate level of nursing skill is available in the immediate postpartum period.

Haemorrhage or circulatory overload causing pulmonary oedema was the cause of death in five women in whom anaesthesia was considered to have contributed to death. The management of severe haemorrhage is a team effort and skilled experienced help may be required particularly in the obstetric patient. Central venous pressure and direct arterial pressure monitoring were not used early enough, or at all, in any of these cases though such monitoring has proved invaluable in managing severe haemorrhage in general surgical or trauma cases. The ready availability of blood and blood products is essential. The transfusion services should be encouraged to include the appropriate quantities of fresh frozen plasma and platelets whenever there is an emergency request for more than five units of blood.

Ischaemic heart disease in women is increasing in prevalence. It should be suspected in women in their thirties or forties if they smoke, have essential hypertension or diabetes. An antenatal ECG in patients who are at risk may be useful. Care should be taken to ensure stability of the heart rate and blood pressure during anaesthesia to avoid subendocardial ischaemia.

Congenital heart disease, whether surgically corrected or not, presents a significant risk since pregnancy and labour produce marked alterations in circulatory dynamics. Careful maintenance of central venous and arterial pressures is essential. The choice between regional or general anaesthesia in congenital heart disease remains controversial and each case should be considered on its merits. Accurate, direct haemodynamic monitoring is indicated whichever technique is used and drugs should be readily available to maintain the circulation.

One death in this triennium was due to an obstructed tracheal tube in a woman being treated with mechanical ventilation and there were five other women in whom substandard postoperative care was considered to have contributed to the death. The anaesthetist is responsible for the patient until full recovery has occurred but cannot be expected to fulfil this obligation if appropriate facilities are not provided.

There should be a designated recovery area of appropriate size situated close to the operating theatre in every obstetric unit in which anaesthetics are given, and patients should remain in this area until they are fully conscious and in a stable cardiorespiratory state. The recovery area should be supervised by the anaesthetic department who should ensure that the nursing staff are trained to deal with the unconscious patient, that adequate therapeutic and monitoring equipment is provided and that there are clear lines or responsibility and delegation. Small units should be capable of providing high dependency care on an occasional basis within such a recovery area. However, larger units dealing with high risk patients with pre-eclampsia or other life-threatening conditions require a high dependency area where skilled nursing can be provided on a one nurse to two patients basis 24 hours a day. Such an area requires equipment for resuscitation together with full facilities for cardiovascular and respiratory monitoring. There should also be equipment for short term ventilatory support pending transfer of the patient to an ICU. The unit may be administered by an anaesthetist or the responsibility may be shared by the anaesthetic and obstetric departments, but again there must be clearly defined lines of responsibility and close liaison between medical and nursing staff.

When patients develop severe complications and it is necessary to transfer them to an intensive care unit it is important to define appropriate lines of communication and for obstetricians and anaesthetists to continue to provide their own specialised input into patient care.

Many of the problems identified in this report were associated with a failure of communication between the obstetrician and anaesthetist. Any woman with a potential problem should be referred to the anaesthetist as soon as this is recognised. If a problem is identified the notes should be 'flagged' with a distinctive label so that all medical and nursing staff are alerted and the anaesthetist can be warned shortly after the woman has been admitted.

References

1. Anonymous. The laryngeal mask: cautionary tales [Correspondence]. Anaesthesia 1990; 45: 167–8.
2. Wee M Y K. The oesophageal detector device. Anaesthesia 1988; 43: 27–9.
3. Nunn J F. The oesophageal detector device. Anaesthesia 1988; 43: 804.
4. Association of Anaesthetists. Recommendations for Standard of Monitoring during Anaesthesia and Recovery. 1988.

CHAPTER 10

Other Direct deaths

Summary

There were 20 Direct deaths from miscellaneous causes, and also two other deaths from air embolism complicating abortion, one spontaneous and one legal, which are counted in Chapter 6. In nine of these the cause of death was clearly established but in 11 cases there was an inadequate or unsatisfactory explanation for the cause of death.

Other Direct deaths

There were 20 Other Direct maternal deaths which have been coded according to the 9th Edition (ICD9) of the International Classification of Diseases, as follows:

ICD 639.9	Sudden death of unknown cause after abortion	1
ICD 646.7	Liver disorders in pregnancy	6
ICD 646.9	Sudden death of unknown cause in pregnancy	5
ICD 648.9	Sudden death of unknown cause in labour	1
ICD 673.0	Obstetric air embolism	1
ICD 674.9	Sudden death of unknown cause in the puerperium	6

Liver diseases

Liver diseases associated with hypertensive disorders of pregnancy are counted and discussed in Chapter 2. There were six deaths associated with acute fatty liver but the clinical presentation varied considerably. The diagnosis was confirmed at autopsy in all but one case, in which autopsy was refused.

Three patients presented with jaundice.

One woman gave a history of infective hepatitis B. She was admitted at term in early labour and was noted to be jaundiced. She had recently been given ampicillin for a urinary tract infection. Caesarean section was performed because of fetal distress. Three hours after delivery she collapsed suddenly, her subsequent death being associated with respiratory failure and disseminated intravascular coagulation (DIC). Acute fatty liver was confirmed at autopsy.

A women, who presented with jaundice, was admitted in labour at 33 weeks gestation, and a Caesarean section was performed because of an oblique lie and twin pregnancy. She developed hepatorenal failure and DIC. There was clearly lack of liaison between obstetricians, physicians and intensive therapists during her subsequent management because the seriousness of her condition was not recognised. A major complicating factor was fluid overload.

A woman of high parity was admitted at 37 weeks gestation with a 'flu-like' illness and jaundice. The initial diagnosis of infective hepatitis was revised to cholestatic jaundice of pregnancy following laboratory investigation which included a negative hepatitis antigen B test. Two days later, after development of DIC, a diagnosis of acute fatty liver was made and a decision was made to deliver the baby. Delivery was by Caesarean section because of fetal distress. As the result of consultation with a haematologist transfusion with coagulation factors was commenced during the Caesarean section. Blood loss was recorded as 1500ml. Postpartum cardiac arrest occurred and was satisfactorily treated. On the second postoperative day the patient was still hypotensive and had by then received a total transfusion of 18 units of blood. A haemoperitoneum was diagnosed and at laparotomy a ruptured spleen was found, the cause of which was unclear. There was no comment on the appearance of the liver. The following day a further laparotomy was performed because of recurrence of haemoperitoneum and the internal iliac arteries were ligated.

Death was primarily the consequence of severe liver dysfunction and coagulopathy. As autopsy was refused the clinical diagnosis of acute yellow atrophy could not be confirmed

In three cases jaundice was a late subsidiary feature and the diagnosis was initially obscure.

A woman, who had multiple endocrinopathy with growth hormone deficiency, hypoparathyriodism and impaired glucose tolerance, was admitted at 33 weeks gestation with polyhydramnios and leg pain, followed by chest pain. A provisional diagnosis of pulmonary embolism was made and she was treated with heparin. Her general condition deteriorated and she was delivered by Caesarean section. She died two weeks postpartum from hepatorenal failure. Histology confirmed acute fatty liver.

A woman was admitted at 34 weeks gestation with a history of nausea. She had proteinuria and glycosuria and also complained of a sore throat. There were reduced fetal movements and a Caesarean section was performed. A liver biopsy was carried out at the same time. Her condition deteriorated postpartum, with hepatic failure and adult respiratory distress syndrome (ARDS). Acute fatty liver of pregnancy was confirmed at autopsy.

A woman was re-admitted two weeks after an uneventful Caesarean section. She had been unwell since the seventh postpartum day and on admission complained of chest pain and dyspnoea and was confused and agitated. The initial differential diagnosis was septicaemia or pulmonary embolism. She was sustained on general supportive therapy and antibiotics but soon developed DIC and renal failure. However her condition deteriorated in spite of haemodialysis. Cholecystitis was suspected and a cholecystectomy was performed. Her condition continued to deteriorate and she died the following day. Acute fatty liver was confirmed at autopsy.

Comment

The number of deaths attributed to acute fatty liver has increased, possibly because of greater awareness of the diagnosis. Ultrasound and computed tomography (CT) scans may assist in the diagnosis but percutaneous liver biopsy is usually contraindicated because of coagulation disorders. These cases emphasise the serious nature of acute fatty liver, which in the past has had a reported mortality rate of the order of 80%, although more recent reports suggest a better prognosis.

DIC creates major difficulties and hazards in management as operative intervention is frequently required. Early consultation with haematologists is essential. Adequate supplies of blood products must be ensured and effective treatment started before initiating any intervention.

Acute fatty liver is more common in areas where there is gross malnutrition, but there was no clear evidence of malnutrition in any of the reported cases, although one had had sickness during the pregnancy which was sufficient to require promazine therapy for a short period. It may also be associated with drugs which depress protein synthesis but the only recorded drug histories were promazine mentioned above and ampicillin for a urinary infection in another case. Only three of the six cases presented with jaundice.

Substandard care

The seriousness of the disorder is not always recognised and there appeared to be an underestimate of this seriousness in two cases, even though they both presented with jaundice.

Pathology

These fatalities underline the highly dangerous nature of gross fatty change in the liver, a specific pathological entity associated with pregnancy as a specific organ lesion, the aetiology remaining obscure.

Air embolism

In this triennium there were three deaths associated with air embolism. Two cases complicated abortion, one legal and one spontaneous, and are counted and discussed in Chapter 6.

The third death was of a woman of short stature, with severe kyphoscoliosis and mild congenital hydrocephalus who had been strongly advised against pregnancy. However she continued with the pregnancy and had severe and progressive respiratory embarrassment necessitating Caesarean section at 29 weeks gestation. Subsequent gross abdominal distension required laparotomy but her condition deteriorated during the operation and she died one hour later. Air embolism was diagnosed at autopsy.

Pathology

Air embolism is often difficult to diagnose with certainty at autopsy and is discussed in Chapter 16.

Deaths without satisfactory explanation

There were 13 deaths in which there was an unsatisfactory or inadequate explanation for the cause of death.

Death following termination of pregnancy

An older woman, a heavy smoker, was apparently recovering satisfactorily from a suction termination. She had regained consciousness. About an hour after completion of the operation, whilst in the recovery area, she had a cardiac arrest and she failed to respond to resuscitation. Blood loss was minimal.

No specific cause for death was found at autopsy, although there was marked coronary atheroma which might have led to sudden cardiac arrhythmia.

Deaths in mid-pregnancy

There were five inadequately explained deaths in mid pregnancy, three of which were associated with inhalation of vomit.

A woman, who was at 21 weeks gestation, screamed whilst making a phone call. The recipient of the phone call went to the house and found her dead. Death was ascribed at autopsy to inhalation of vomit but the cause of the vomiting was not identified. She had had blackouts several years previously. There was no other evidence of epilepsy.

A woman died following inhalation of vomit at 28 weeks gestation. She had been found unconscious, lying with her head in the bath, but with no water in the bath. It was reported that she had previously experienced blackouts during the pregnancy. No relevant underlying pathology was identified from the clinical notes and the only finding at autopsy was pyelonephritis.

A teenage girl with a concealed full-term pregnancy was found unconscious and cyanosed in bed, having come home from work saying that she felt sick. She was surrounded by vomit but no stomach contents were found in the respiratory tract. Death was ascribed at autopsy to adult respiratory distress syndrome (ARDS) associated with septicaemia and acute pyelonephritis. Unfortunately no microbiological examinations on body fluids or kidneys were performed.

One woman died following inhalation of vomit at 29 weeks gestation. She lived alone and the evidence suggested that the vomiting was self induced. This case is further discussed in Chapter 16.

A woman at 14 weeks gestation collapsed suddenly during intercourse and had severe vaginal bleeding. It was thought that she had a cerebral vascular accident but there was no evidence of this on CT scan. An extensive autopsy was performed which confirmed the negative CT findings. There was separation of the placenta but the pregnancy sac was intact. There was no evidence of a cerebral accident or any other significant pathology.

Intrapartum death

One woman died during the first stage of labour. Labour was induced because of mild hypertension, starting with *Syntocinon* infusion in conventional dosage. Artificial rupture of the membranes was performed at 6cm cervical dilation. One hour later sudden cardiorespiratory failure developed which failed to respond to prompt and intensive resuscitative measures. A live child, which subsequently died, was delivered by post-mortem Caesarean section. A provisional clinical diagnosis of amniotic fluid embolism was made. In spite of the strong clinical impression no evidence of amniotic fluid embolism (or other cause for her sudden collapse) was identified at autopsy.

Immediate postpartum deaths

There were two deaths immediately postpartum, probably arising from events in labour.

An older woman of high parity who had had previous Caesarean sections had a cervical cerclage performed in the current pregnancy. She was admitted at 26 weeks gestation when it was thought that her membranes had ruptured and the cervical suture was removed. Labour commenced spontaneously one week later and the fetus was born in an intact sac. Immediately following delivery she had respiratory arrest, fits and ventricular fibrillation. She rapidly developed DIC and a clinical diagnosis of amniotic fluid embolism was made. She died shortly afterwards before further treatment could be instituted. A detailed autopsy and histological examination failed to reveal any evidence of amniotic fluid embolism and the cause of death remained obscure.

A parous woman had a twin pregnancy and the first twin was delivered uneventfully as an assisted breech. She had declined epidural anaesthesia. The second twin remained high and there was thought to be possible placental separation with a closed cervix. It was decided to perform a Caesarean section. The junior obstetrician, whilst awaiting the arrival of an anaesthetist, administered salbutamol intravenously to reduce uterine activity. General anaesthesia was induced but the patient had significant tachycardia. Following delivery of the baby the patient developed severe hypotension and cardiac arrest.

There is doubt about the actual cause of death in this case though it is probable that after induction of anaesthesia the cardiac output was compromised due to the large dose of salbutamol causing tachycardia and arteriolar vasodilatation, possibly combined with some aortocaval compression. The combination of severe sympathetic stimulation and general anaesthesia was considered the direct cause of death.

Late postpartum deaths

There were four incompletely explained postpartum deaths.

A woman was found dead in a bathroom with her head in the water three days after a normal delivery. Death was due to drowning but there had also been inhalation of gastric contents. The reason for her collapse was not determined.

It was assumed that the precipitating event was vasovagal syncope but there was no obvious cause for this, although the patient was kneeling over the side of the bath.

A young woman had a normal delivery and returned home on the third postpartum day. On the fourth day she collapsed and had difficulty in breathing and subsequently complained of headaches. She was well by the evening but soon after going to bed screamed and was unable to breathe. At autopsy a provisional diagnosis of cardiomyopathy was made, but could not be supported histologically, so the diagnosis must remain obscure.

A young woman had been delivered by Caesarean section. Forty two days postpartum she collapsed whilst dancing. A full autopsy revealed no cause for the sudden death but no microbiological investigations were carried out.

Possibly death was associated with cardiac arrhythmia for it was noted that, during general anaesthesia for the Caesarean section, she had multiple ventricular ectopics which required administration of lignocaine.

Another young woman had an emergency Caesarean section performed for prolapsed cord shortly after admission to hospital, the membranes having been ruptured for 12 hours. She remained well until her fourth postoperative day when her condition deteriorated, with a clinical picture of septicaemia although she was apyrexial and cultures of blood, urine and lochia were negative. No improvement occurred despite intensive IV therapy. Her condition became worse and it was thought there was intraperitoneal bleeding. A laparotomy was performed and profuse abdominal wall haemorrhages noted, but there was no intraperitoneal bleeding. The clinical picture thereafter was that of a gram negative septicaemia with afibrinogenaemia, and she died two days after the laparotomy. The cultures taken at the time of the laparotomy were negative. The autopsy did not reveal a cause of death. This case is also discussed in Chapter 16.

Pathology

These obscure deaths by definition defy pathological explanation, but diagnoses stand or fall by the quality of the autopsies and the extensiveness of ancillary investigations such as histology and microbiology. Two of the sudden deaths were clinically ascribed to amniotic fluid embolism, but no squames were visible in extensive histological searches of lung tissue.

These deaths, without satisfactory explanation, some with evidence of cardiac arrhythmias, indicate the deficiencies of even the most meticulous autopsies where the fatal lesion is functional rather than morphologically demonstrable. Caution must be employed in blaming terminal phenomena such as 'aspiration of vomit' as the definitive underlying cause of death.

The unexplained intrapartum death illustrates the frequent gap between a seemingly clear cut clinical diagnosis of a condition, such as amniotic fluid embolism, and the lack of supportive evidence at a detailed autopsy.

CHAPTER 11

Cardiac disease

Summary

This chapter details 23 cases of cardiac disease, which in this triennium ranks third after pulmonary embolism and hypertensive disorders as a cause of maternal death. Twenty two deaths were considered to be Indirect. There was one Direct death from Cardiomyopathy. There were also two other women with cardiac disease whose deaths were considered to be Fortuitous and are counted in Chapter 14. Two deaths which were secondary to anaesthesia in high risk patients are counted in Chapter 9. In addition a woman with complete heart block and a pacemaker died of intestinal obstruction and is counted in Chapter 12, as her death was unrelated to her cardiac condition.

Dominant features in the group as a whole are the number of women (six) who proceeded with a pregnancy against strong medical advice; the number of occasions (eight) when the severity and implications of the disease appear to have been underestimated, resulting in lack of team co-operation and inappropriate management; and, as has been emphasised in previous reports, the especially high risk period immediately postpartum.

The number of deaths from congenital heart disease has increased and the proportion of congenital heart disease deaths has also increased, from 22% in 1970–81 to 35% in 1982–84 in England and Wales, and 43% in the United Kingdom in 1985–87.

The increased number of deaths from congenital heart disease is also reflected in the proportion of young mothers (30% under the age of 25 years compared with 24% in 1970–84 in England and Wales) and of primipara (38% compared with 22% in 1970–84).

Cardiac disease also poses special anaesthetic problems which are discussed in Chapter 9.

Cardiac disease

Congenital heart disease

Table 11.1 shows the number of maternal deaths from congenital and acquired heart disease during the six triennia from 1970 to 1987 in England and Wales compared with those in the UK in 1985–1987.

There were 10 deaths in women due to complications of congenital heart disease. One woman who had a congenital narrowing of the left coronary

Table 11.1 *Number of maternal deaths from congenital and acquired cardiac diseases England and Wales during 1970−87 compared with United Kingdom 1985−87.*

		Congenital	Acquired			Total
		Number	Other	Ischaemic	Number	
England & Wales	1970−72	9	N/A	N/A	33	42
	1973−75	4	N/A	N/A	14	18
	1976−78	3	N/A	N/A	14	17
	1979−81	4	6	6	12	16
	1982−84	6	3	8	11	17
	1985−87	10	3	6	9	19
United Kingdom	1985−87	10	4	9	13	23

artery and died following an infarction, is described under 'Ischaemic heart disease'. A death due to complications of anaesthesia in a patient with pulmonary hypertension is counted in Chapter 9.

In six cases there was a clear record of strong medical advice against pregnancy or continuing with the pregnancy.

Five women had previous surgery for anatomical defects but all suffered continuing cardiac disability. The other five cases had primary pulmonary hypertension.

Deaths during pregnancy

Four deaths (including the case described under 'ischaemic heart disease') occurred during pregnancy.

One was a woman with complex anomalies who had had cardiac surgery on two occasions and had a history of Q fever, endocarditis, hepatitis and nephrotic syndrome. She was first seen with infective endocarditis when she was 18 weeks pregnant and died shortly afterwards in spite of expert management.

Another death occurred in early pregnancy, in a woman who had had surgical treatment for ventricular septal defect and valvular heart disease and several attacks of infective endocarditis, including one early in the current pregnancy. She had a mid-trimester spontaneous abortion and was admitted one week later with severe dyspnoea and in congestive cardiac failure. Emergency heart surgery was attempted but the patient died on the operating table as a result of aorto-ventricular disconnection. No autopsy was carried out.

A woman with Eisenmenger's syndrome had been strongly advised against pregnancy but refused termination. At 33 weeks gestation she felt unwell, was admitted to hospital and died in her sleep the same night. Autopsy revealed cardiac tamponade associated with rupture of a pulmonary artery aneurysm.

Deaths during labour or immediately after labour

Six patients died during labour or immediately afterwards, as did the case of pulmonary hypertension counted in Chapter 9.

A young primigravida with Eisenmenger's syndrome collapsed immediately after a forceps delivery under epidural analgesia. Intensive resuscitative measures were of only temporary effect and final cardiac arrest occurred 19 hours after delivery.

Another young primigravida, with residual pulmonary hypertension after open-heart surgery for Eisenmenger's syndrome was delivered with forceps under epidural analgesia and collapsed during the third stage with acute pulmonary oedema. The choice of anesthesia in such cases is discussed in Chapter 9.

A woman with severe primary pulmonary hypertension had a normal labour with epidural analgesia. When in advanced labour she became cyanotic and her blood pressure fell. This was rapidly followed by acute right ventricular failure and cardiac arrest.

Certain features of her care were considered to be substandard, and it would have been preferable for her to be delivered in an obstetric unit close to a cardiology centre.

A woman with an aortic valve prosthesis developed bacterial endocarditis and was delivered as an emergency by Caesarean section at 33 weeks gestation. There was valvular detachment and embolisation immediately postpartum.

Whilst consultation between the obstetricians and the anaesthetists had taken place, the decision was taken to anaesthetise the patient in the obstetric unit. In retrospect it would have been preferable, knowing the high risk and possible need for emergency cardiac surgery, to have performed the Caesarean section in a unit with appropriate facilities and staff for emergency surgery.

A highly parous woman with pulmonary hypertension developed acute dyspnoea, orthopnoea and hypotension at 33 weeks gestation. She went into spontaneous labour at that time and had an assisted breech delivery in the intensive care unit (ICU). Cardiac arrest occurred thirty minutes postpartum.

A woman with severe primary pulmonary hypertension, who had been strongly advised against pregnancy, did not accept advice to stay in hospital during the antenatal period. She had spontaneous delivery following a nine hour labour, with a blood loss of 250ml. She collapsed suddenly five minutes postpartum.

Care was considered substandard partly because of lack of patient co-operation but also lack of professional team work, despite there being plenty of time available to make appropriate arrangements. Only an obstetric registrar was present at the delivery. There was also lack of detail in the autopsy report.

Puerperal death

There was only one death which occurred later in the puerperium.

A woman with undiagnosed pulmonary hypertension, whose only recognised medical disability was chronic urinary tract infection, was delivered by elective Caesarean section because of breech presentation and poor fetal growth. The early puerperium was uneventful but she collapsed suddenly on the twenty-third day postpartum. She was admitted to hospital but resuscitation was unavailing.

There was lack of detail in the autopsy report but histology showed features characteristic of pulmonary hypertension. Blood cultures taken at the time of death failed to grow any pathogens.

Acquired heart disease

Table 11.2 shows the number of maternal deaths from acquired heart disease by age for the six triennia from 1970 to 1987 for England and Wales, compared with the UK for 1985–87.

Table 11.2 *Number of maternal deaths from acquired cardiac disease, by age, for England and Wales 1970–87 compared with the United Kingdom 1985–87.*

		Age (years)				
		Under 25	25–29	30–34	35 and over	Total
England & Wales	1970–72	8	6	4	15	33
	1973–75	3	5	1	5	14
	1976–78	5	3	1	5	14
	1979–81	4	1	2	5	12
	1982–84	0	2	4	5	11
	1985–87	2	0	4	3	9
United Kingdom	1985–87	2	1	6	4	13

Ischaemic heart disease

There were nine deaths associated with ischaemic heart disease. Five occurred during the antenatal period and four postpartum.

Although three deaths were in women over the age of 40 years there were two deaths in the third decade and four in the fourth decade. In two cases there was evidence of substandard care. The first was failure to recognise that the woman had stopped taking anticoagulants and the other was failure to carry out an electrocardiogram (ECG) before Caesarean section.

Antepartum deaths

In three cases death occurred before twelve weeks gestation.

A young cigarette smoker, who took oral contraceptives for over five years, developed chest pain at 11 weeks gestation but did not seek advice and collapsed suddenly a few days later. She had coronary atheroma with complete occlusion of the left main artery. Her lipids were normal.

A young woman of high parity was a heavy cigarette smoker. She gave a history of chest pain in previous pregnancies. She was admitted through the Accident and Emergency Department at eight weeks gestation complaining of chest pain. Cardiac arrest occurred whilst an ECG was being organised. Autopsy showed coronary atheroma and thrombosis.

A woman had been treated for hypertension, hyperthyroidism and peripheral vascular disease which required femoro-popliteal angioplasty. She had been prescribed warfarin but had discontinued it. She was admitted to an ICU as an emergency in early pregnancy and found to have an anterior infarction. She died five days later and no autopsy was carried out.

Although this woman had been seen by a general practitioner and an obstetrician neither had elicited the history of discontinued anticoagulant therapy. This was probably an aetiological factor, so must be regarded as substandard care.

An older woman died at 33 weeks gestation. She had an attack of chest pain at home but cardiac arrest had occurred by the time of her admission. Autopsy showed minimal atherosis but a dissecting aneurysm of the left main stem coronary artery with compression of the lumen.

Another woman died suddenly in the second trimester. Death was due to coronary thrombosis associated with congenital narrowing of the left coronary artery. There was also evidence of previous infarction. In her first pregnancy she had chest pain in mid-pregnancy but no cardiac abnormality was found and her symptoms were ascribed to reflux oesophagitis.

Postpartum Deaths

An elderly grand multipara was hypertensive and had gestational diabetes. She went into labour at 35 weeks gestation and had a Caesarean section after five hours in labour. Cardiac arrest occurred immediately after delivery, and she died despite resuscitative measures. Autopsy showed coronary atheroma and occlusion.

In spite of this history she did not have a preoperative ECG examination and this was regarded as substandard care.

Another elderly multiparous woman was anaemic, overweight and a heavy cigarette smoker. She was delivered by Caesarean section at 36 weeks gestation because of placenta praevia, with a blood loss of approximately 1 litre. Postoperatively she developed left ventricular failure, and cardiac arrest occurred three hours after delivery. Autopsy showed severe coronary atheroma and calcification.

A parous woman, overweight and a heavy smoker on oral contraception immediately prior to pregnancy, had an uneventful spontaneous delivery and was discharged home the next day. Shortly after her discharge she had chest pain which was attributed to hyperventilation associated with anxiety. However about two weeks later she collapsed suddenly and died. Autopsy showed thrombotic occlusion of the coronary artery and several infarcts of at least one week's duration.

One older woman who had a normal delivery, had a postpartum illness initially diagnosed as chest infection. This was revised later to cardiomyopathy when her condition deteriorated in the early puerperium and a heart transplant was carried out. However there were signs of rejection and cardiac arrest two days later. Histology of the patient's own heart showed left main coronary artery atheroma with almost complete occlusion of the lumen, and no evidence of cardiomyopathy.

Other cardiac deaths

There were four other deaths from cardiac disease counted in this section. Three of these patients were at high risk with medical problems. One was a Direct death from cardiomyopathy. There was also a death associated with epidural anaesthesia, in a patient who had aortic incompetence, which is described in Chapter 9.

An older woman had had two previous cerebral infarcts associated with rheumatic heart disease and had been advised strongly against pregnancy. Valvotomy had been performed. In mid-pregnancy she developed gastroenteritis and this was followed by infective endocarditis.

Her care was considered to be substandard, partly because she refused to accept medical advice and partly because the help of a cardiologist had not been sought until she was admitted in cardiac failure.

A young primigravida developed tonsillitis and a heart murmur was noted. She was seen by a physician who considered that there was no abnormality. She was admitted at 33 weeks gestation in labour and suffered a small abruption. She was delivered with forceps, without anaesthesia. She became dyspnoeic during delivery and was transferred to the intensive care unit but failed to respond to treatment. She was found at autopsy to have infective endocarditis.

A multiparous woman had an incomplete mid-trimester abortion; she was shocked at the time of admission and her haemoglobin concentration was only 6.8g/dl. Manual removal of the placenta was carried out under general anaesthesia and she was transferred to the ICU. On the third day she became dyspnoeic and was thought to have a pulmonary embolism. Cardiac arrest occurred during insertion of a pulmonary artery catheter. The chest was opened to explore for embolism and to carry out embolectomy but no embolus was found. Death was ascribed to myocarditis of unknown aetiology.

Another woman developed cough and dyspnoea in late pregnancy. She had an uneventful delivery but her symptoms increased postpartum and were initially attributed to respiratory disease. On the 9th postpartum day an ECG showed right heart preponderance; her condition deteriorated and she died the following day. Autopsy showed cardiomyopathy.

Treatment was delayed and inappropriate because of delay in diagnosis — not uncommon because of the non-specific symptoms associated with this condition, which should always be considered in the differential diagnosis of cardiac failure in the puerperium.

Substandard care

The dominant factor in cases where care was considered substandard was the failure of the patient to accept advice (seven cases). On the medical side, lack of team consultation, too late involvement of colleagues, and delivery in circumstances inadequate to cope with major complications, all contributed to substandard care.

Discussion

Problems associated with congenital heart disease have been highlighted in this triennium. Although, following surgery, many patients appear relatively fit their cardiovascular system does not cope readily with the additional load of pregnancy and, especially, labour. Their apparent fitness makes them reluctant to accept medical advice against becoming pregnant and also tends to mislead their medical attendants.

Epidural analgesia and general anaesthesia pose a number of problems especially in patients with intracardiac shunts.

The need for early involvement of cardiologist and anaesthetists with the obstetricians in a team approach, preferably at combined clinics, again needs emphasis. In general, because of the need for close consultant supervision and continuity, antenatal care shared with the general practitioner is inappropriate. Careful consideration also needs to be given to the place of delivery.

Because of the acute problems which may arise, a formal plan of management should be agreed and written in the notes so that duty staff can act promptly in an emergency. Patients having a Caesarean section, especially those who have had previous cardiac surgery, should be delivered in a unit where appropriate facilities and staff are available for management of any cardiac surgical emergency. If necessary the obstetric and neonatal team should be prepared to provide facilities in the Cardiac Unit.

Pathology

The cardiac deaths show a diversity of causes with no common pathological thread. Coronary artery disease contributed over a third of the fatalities, the majority occurring under the age of 40 years. Cardiomyopathy seems under-represented compared to the general population, especially in a young adult group such as this. Infective endocarditis remains a problem, even with the extensive armoury of antibiotics now available.

Several cases with no clear-cut postmortem diagnoses emphasise the need for adequate histology after autopsy, with multiple blocks available for study.

Addendum

The case report for one young woman who died of cardiomyopathy un-delivered, at 28 weeks gestation arrived too late to be included in the main tables and discussion. She was a Direct obstetric death. There were minimal clinical details, although autopsy revealed cardiomyopathy with hypertrophy of the left ventricle. No other abnormality was detected.

CHAPTER 12

Other Indirect causes of maternal death

Contents	Page

Summary

There were 84 Indirect deaths representing 30% of all Direct and Indirect deaths compared with 34% for England and Wales in the last triennium. Twenty-two were deaths from cardiac disease described in Chapter 11; the remaining 62 deaths are discussed in this Chapter.

Definition

Indirect maternal deaths are defined as those resulting from a previously existing disease, or disease that developed during pregnancy and which did not have a Direct obstetric cause, but which was aggravated by the physiological effects of pregnancy. This definition has also been interpreted here to include deaths in which the pre-existing disease resulted in significant changes in the treatment or management of the pregnancy, or of the condition itself, eg diabetes, epilepsy.

Classification of cases

In the chapter the cases have been grouped according to the International Classification of Diseases, Injuries and Causes of Death (revision ICD 9), except for 'Sudden unnatural deaths', which have been grouped according to the inquest verdicts of the coroner or procurator fiscal rather than to the cause of death (eg to 'suicide' rather than 'overdose' or 'hanging').

A separate contents list of the ICD headings (see page 103) has been included for ease of reference.

i. Infectious diseases

There were ten Indirect deaths which were considered to be related to infectious diseases, four of which were related to respiratory complications of chicken pox, one to a rare respiratory infection and five from other infections.

a. *Chicken Pox (Varicella)*

One young parous woman para 2, was admitted at 38 weeks gestation with chicken pox and bronchopneumonia. She also had a urinary tract infection due to *beta-haemolytic streptococcus*. She developed adult respiratory distress syndrome (ARDS), disseminated intravascular coagulation (DIC) and acute renal failure from which she never recovered. Although there was a detailed autopsy there was no specific comment on whether or not viral inclusion bodies were found in the histological sections.

The second parous woman was admitted to an intensive care unit (ICU) with a varicella pneumonitis at 27 weeks gestation. Her respiratory difficulties became extreme and it was decided to deliver her by Caesarean section because of fetal distress. It was also hoped that the maternal ventilation would improve, but her respiratory condition deteriorated and she died in the fourth week after delivery, the day after a laparotomy was carried out for suspected intestinal obstruction. Autopsy was refused, but virology studies had confirmed the clinical diagnosis of varicella pneumonia.

The third woman, also parous, was admitted with chicken pox and varicella bronchopneumonia at 27 weeks gestation. She had a spontaneous delivery at 28 weeks with a rapid progression to respiratory failure. She was ventilated for four days prior to her death from DIC and acute renal failure. Autopsy confirmed the diagnosis of bronchopneumonia and pox marks were present on the trachea.

A fourth woman of high parity had varicella pneumonia at 31 weeks gestation. She went into premature labour at 32 weeks. Her respiratory condition became worse and she developed DIC and acute renal failure, dying 11 hours after delivery. No autopsy was performed.

b. *Infection due to Mycobacterium-aveum-intracellular-scrofulaceum.*

A primigravid woman died from an unusual respiratory infection super-imposed on progressive cardiac failure. This was primarily related to con-structive pericarditis as a consequence of high dosage mediastinal radio-therapy and aggressive chemotherapy for a reticulum cell sarcoma. This had involved the right lung, chest wall and sternum 15 years previously.

At 27 weeks gestation she had a diaphragmatic pleurisy and chest infection. Sputum cultures grew acid-fast bacilli, and anti-tuberculous therapy was commenced. The chest infection appeared to be improving when she developed signs of right heart failure. A clinical diagnosis of pericardial tamponade/constrictive pericarditis was made and she was transferred to a cardiothoracic unit. During an emergency thoracotomy massive bleeding occurred when an attempt was made to elevate the sternum from the dense adhesions from her previous radiotherapy and the patient never recovered.

The progressive cardiac failure was primarily related to constrictive peri-carditis, a consequence of previous radiotherapy and chemotherapy. The increased cardiac load of pregnancy and the pulmonary infection undoubt-edly precipitated the fatal sequence of events. Even with the detailed autopsy and microbiological report it is difficult to be certain which was more important. The success of the treatment of the malignancy was a factor in relation to this woman's subsequent pregnancy. However, the acid-fast bacilli were considered to be pathogenic by the consultant micro-biologists involved. For this reason this death has been counted as Indirect.

c. *Other infections*

There were five other cases, all of which had deficiencies in the clinical and/or autopsy details and summary of the cases. They were all considered to have substandard aspects.

There was a young woman who had a streptococcal septicaemia, which probably started in the upper respiratory tract. Following her emergency admission with an inevitable abortion the severity of the rapid and over-whelming infection was not appreciated. She died within 12 hours of her admission. The diagnosis was made on the results of antemortem and postmortem bacteriological tests rather than on a limited and sub-standard autopsy.

The second parous woman, who was afraid of dental treatment, was admitted as an emergency at 35 weeks gestation with severe Ludwig's angina and septicaemia secondary to a submandibular abscess. Following this she went into a spontaneous labour of short duration and had a forceps delivery in the intensive care unit (ICU) under full mechanical ventilation. Her respiratory difficulties continued in conjunction with a severe septicaemia and she died two weeks after her admission. No autopsy was performed.

The third parous woman had vomiting and failure to gain weight throughout her pregnancy. Although she had persistent vomiting and headaches it was not considered that she had a physical cause for her symptoms and was predominantly under the care of the psychiatric team. She had a forceps delivery after the spontaneous onset of labour. Four days after delivery she had a fit and investigations showed tuberculous meningitis, also confirmed at autopsy. This case illustrates the danger of labelling a patient as anxious or pyschotic before eliminating a physical cause for symptoms.

The fourth case was that of a parous woman who returned from holiday abroad with Hepatitis B infection. She had a mid-trimester spontaneous abortion at 16 weeks gestation. Following evacuation of retained products without anaesthesia a laparotomy was required for intraperitoneal bleeding from the pelvic sidewall. She died one day after delivery. Autopsy was refused by the family on religious grounds but a postmortem liver sample confirmed the diagnosis of Hepatitis B.

The final case was of a young woman who had a severe infection of the right eye which was treated with tetracycline. She refused admission on two occasions. Her condition deteriorated and at 29 weeks gestation she delivered a stillbirth secondary to septicaemia at home, and was then admitted to hospital. She had a worsening orbital cellulitis and investigations revealed intracranial collections of pus and severe pan-sinusitis. Despite two operations to remove the pus and drain the sinuses and intensive antibiotic therapy, her condition deteriorated. She died in the second week after delivery. Autopsy revealed extensive intracranial infection with widespread cortical thrombophlebitis. There was no postmortem microbiological or detailed histological information.

ii. Neoplastic diseases

There were four Indirect deaths from neoplasm as compared with 11 in England and Wales in the last triennium. In no case was there substandard care.

The first death was that of a multiparous woman who had a normal pregnancy and delivery. From the first day of the puerperium she felt increasingly unwell and initially a diagnosis of endometritis was made. On the third day a full biochemical scan revealed hypercalcaemia with uraemia and hyperparathyroidism was diagnosed. The skull X-ray showed 'pepperpot' changes and abdominal X-ray showed calcinosis in both kidneys. Despite expert care in the ICU her condition deteriorated and she died in the first week of the puerperium. Just prior to death a parathyroid adenoma, which was the primary cause of death, was removed.

The second case was a woman who died from a phaeochromocytoma shortly after delivery of her first child by Caesarean section. She was booked early in the antenatal clinic, with a 20 year history of paroxysmal tachycardia, for which she had been admitted two years prior to this pregnancy with a blood pressure of 180/90 mm Hg and a pulse rate of

180 beats per minute. Her blood pressure never rose above 135/90 mm Hg. She was found to have an abnormal glucose tolerance test at 35 weeks gestation and had a technically difficult delivery by Caesarean section of a baby weighing 5.3kg with much bleeding from the uterine incision. Postoperatively there was dyspnoea and tachycardia followed shortly by a cardiac arrest. Although the heart was restarted and she was moved to the ICU, death occurred a few hours later. The rapid death was due to acute myocardial failure secondary to the phaeo-chromocytoma; the case is also discussed in Chapter 9. Apart from the history before pregnancy, the presentation was rather atypical of phaeochromocytoma.

The third case involved a young woman, who at the time she became pregnant, was known to have a spinal tumour. At 32 weeks gestation the neurosurgeons decided that removal was essential if paraplegia was to be avoided. A haemangioblastoma was removed successfully after a long surgical procedure with the patient lying prone, but unfortunately she died the next day from a pulmonary embolus.

The fourth case was a young multiparous woman who was a known epileptic. During early pregnancy her epilepsy became difficult to control despite regular anticonvulsant medication. At 25 weeks gestation she developed excessive vomiting and lower abdominal pain with episodes of hypoglycaemia and abnormal liver function tests. A month later she was transferred to a teaching hospital where a Caesarean section was performed because of fetal distress, and deposits of secondary adeno-carcinoma were found throughout the abdomen. Her condition worsened and she died about three weeks later. A coroner's autopsy failed to reveal the origin of the primary carcinoma. This case is of interest because of the bizarre clinical presentation during the second trimester in a previously healthy young woman. There was no substandard care.

iii. Endocrine, nutritional, metabolic and immunity disorders.

There were six cases in one of whom was care substandard.

a. *Diabetes mellitus*

A parous woman was known to have had diabetes for many years complicated by retinopathy and hyperthyroidism. She booked early with a blood pressure of 110/70 mm Hg and clear urine. She controlled her diabetes poorly and, because of proteinuria and mild hypertension she was admitted to the consultant unit in mid-pregnancy. At 26 weeks she suffered a transient right-sided hemiparesis. She was also noted to have ischaemic changes on the ECG, with enlargement of the left ventricle thought to be due to cardiomyopathy. Labour was induced prior to term for fetal growth retardation and a baby weighing 2.38kg was delivered. Six days later she was sent home apparently well, but was readmitted the following day with weakness of the left arm and leg thought to be due to a cerebral infarction. She died in the fourth postnatal week. Autopsy was refused.

A young woman, an insulin dependent diabetic, was also known to have died eight days after an emergency Caesarean section for fetal distress. Only the autopsy report was made available to the enquiry which revealed that she died from *Staphylococcus Aureus* bronchopneumonia.

b. *Autoimmune disease*

A woman who was only a few weeks pregnant gave a two day history of feeling unwell.

A diagnosis of 'hyperemesis of pregnancy' was made by the general practitioner. A short while after seeing him the patient collapsed and died from what, at autopsy, was shown to be an Addisonian crisis with autoimmune adrenalitis and pericarditis.

c. *Anaphylactic reaction*

A parous woman with asthma but a normal obstetric history was seen on four occasions in the antenatal clinic before the diagnosis of iron-deficiency anaemia with a haemoglobin concentration of 8.6g/dl was made. It was decided she should be treated with intramuscular *Imferon*. In view of the recognised risk of anaphylactic reactions associated with this compound and the fact that the patient was an asthmatic, a resuscitation trolley was placed next to her. Following the administration of 5 ml of *Imferon* acute bronchospasm developed. Cortisone 200mg, and *Piriton* 10mg, were given intravenously and adrenaline (1:1,000) 1 ml was given intradermally, but to no avail. Despite immediate transfer to the ICU death occurred 30 hours later.

This case illustrates the importance of avoiding a potentially dangerous course of management, such as intramuscular iron for treatment of a moderate iron-deficiency anaemia without a test dose, when there are still 14 weeks of pregnancy before term. Even though such management does not always result in a return of the haemoglobin concentration to normal levels the risks during pregnancy and labour of such an anaemia are small.

d. *Lupus erythematosus*

A young woman was known to have systemic lupus erythematosus (SLE) involving the brain, kidneys and lungs. In view of this she was admitted to the consultant unit for rest from 15 weeks gestation. Her hypertension proved difficult to control and a few weeks later she had a cardiac arrest from which she was successfully resuscitated. The following week she had a hysterotomy for uncontrollable bleeding. Her condition deteriorated and she died two weeks after the operation. At autopsy, although death was considered to have been from hypertensive heart disease, several old cerebral infarcts were found in addition to numerous unruptured berry aneurysms unrelated to the SLE.

e. *Acute pancreatitis*

A 29 year old parous woman had a vaginal delivery at full-term. She complained of left sided chest pain later the same day and early the following day. No abnormal signs were found. A few hours later her abdomen became distended and a diagnosis of acute pancreatitis was made, confirmed by a grossly elevated serum amylase. She was transferred to the ICU for intensive conservative and supportive measures over the next week. In face of a deteriorating situation it was decided to perform a laparotomy, but cardiac arrest prevented this. Autopsy confirmed the diagnosis of acute pancreatitis with extensive fat necrosis.

Since acute pancreatitis is so uncommon at this age it is considered that this must be regarded as an Indirect death.

iv. Blood diseases

There was one case of sickle-cell disease.

The case involved a multiparous African woman known to have homozygous sickle-cell disease. Antenatal care was uneventful and she was admitted at term in spontaneous labour. A pre-arranged plan had been drawn up by the consultant for the management of labour and all went well until acute fetal distress developed, necessitating delivery by Caesarean section. Unfortunately the first day of her puerperium was complicated by a chest infection which led to a sickle-cell crisis. She was transferred to a teaching hospital and an exchange transfusion was performed. She had artificial ventilation for adult respiratory distress syndrome (ARDS) but she died in the third postpartum week.

This case illustrates the dangers of homozygous sickle-cell disease however good the standard of clinical care in the unit. It seems sensible to plan for delivery of these cases in a centre with special expertise in caring for the condition.

v. Mental disorders

Alcohol and/or drug dependency

There were two cases, in both of which the care was substandard.

The first case involved a parous woman with an eight-year history of alcoholism complicated by sideroblastic anaemia and peripheral neuritis. She was admitted to hospital without prior antenatal care at 26 weeks gestation draining offensive liquor from which a *beta-haemolytic streptococcus* was grown. Having had a rigor, she was treated with antibiotics and delivered a stillborn baby with multiple malformations two hours later. She went home after an uneventful puerperium, having been given *Depo-Provera* for contraception. Nineteen days after delivery she suddenly dropped dead whilst talking to a friend. At autopsy death was thought to be due to acute left ventricular failure secondary to a cardiomyopathy. However the precise diagnosis must remain in doubt because of a substandard autopsy with no histology of the myocardium and in the absence of cirrhosis. The failure to attend for antenatal care is considered to have been substandard care on the part of the patient.

In the second case a woman with a history of alcoholism booked early in pregnancy and then attended only once for antenatal care. At 32 weeks gestation she was admitted unconscious to hospital and smelling of alcohol, but took her own discharge as soon as she regained consciousness. Blood taken for toxicity tests was not analysed despite the admission by the patient that she had taken some form of tablets prior to admission. Two days later she was readmitted with an intrauterine infection and a dead fetus. Labour was induced by *Syntocinon* and a normal delivery resulted. Shortly afterwards she started to hallucinate, became unconscious and some hours later she had a cardiac arrest. A coroner's autopsy revealed that death was due to paracetamol hepatotoxicity and alcohol intoxication.

There is evidence of substandard care in three aspects of the management. The general practice staff, with whom she booked, failed to notice that she only came back once for antenatal care and no attempt was made to follow her up. Then, on the first hospital admission, the medical staff failed to pursue the possibility of drug overdose in a patient who came in unconscious. Finally, some blame must attach to the patient for her behaviour throughout the pregnancy which ultimately contributed to her death.

vi. Diseases of the central nervous system

a. *Intracranial haemorrhage*

There were 15 deaths from intracranial haemorrhage, and one death from cerebral infarction resulting from carotid artery thrombosis. Two women had hypertension but 13 deaths were unrelated to hypertensive disorders.

Table 12.1 *Deaths from intracranial haemorrhage.*

Description	Number of cases
Diagnosis confirmed by autopsy	5
Berry aneurysm	3
Cavernous haemangioma	1
Vascular malformation	1
No autopsy (4 had organs removed for transplantation) Diagnosis by:	6
CT scan	3
Angiography	1
Lumbar puncture	1
Craniotomy	1
Described in text	4
Confirmed by craniotomy	1
Uncertain causes	3
Total	15

In only five instances was the source of bleeding identified at autopsy. In three cases subarachnoid haemorrhage was due to rupture of a berry aneurysm. In one it was due to the rupture of a cavernous haemangioma in the posterior part of the pons and in the other case there was a confirmed vascular malformation, but its precise site not stated. Four of these women collapsed and became unconscious antenatally. In one woman there had been a preceding fit.

110

No autopsy was performed in six cases. Four of these women had organs taken for transplantation. The diagnosis was made by CT scan in three cases and by angiography, lumbar puncture and at craniotomy respectively in each of the others.

Seven of these 11 women had either headaches, or a fit or collapsed and became unconscious before the onset of labour, and it is considered that the physiological changes of pregnancy had been an aggravating factor.

With regard to the other four women:

The first woman, who was admitted semi-comatose at 33 weeks gestation, had a craniotomy for cerebral haemorrhage. As her condition deteriorated an emergency Caesarean section was performed, but she died shortly afterwards.

The second woman, a poorly controlled diabetic with diabetic retinitis and cardiomyopathy, had severe headache and weakness of the left arm and leg about two weeks after delivery. Investigations suggested cerebral infarction and she died a week later. Permission for an autopsy was refused. It was impossible to establish whether the cerebrovascular accident was due to atheroma as a consequence of her diabetes or thrombosis associated with pregnancy. The death, in this instance, has been coded to cerebral haemorrhage and included in this section.

The third woman collapsed in the third stage of labour following a normal delivery and postpartum haemorrhage. After resuscitation she was transferred to the ICU of another hospital. A CT scan revealed a large intracerebral mass with hydrocephalus and she was pronounced brain stem dead later the same day. It was initially felt that the woman had died from a brain tumour, but further review of the histology of the brain only revealed evidence of haemorrhage into the cerebellum for which no pathological explanation was identified.

An older woman had a cone biopsy early in pregnancy. She had a late rise in blood pressure in pregnancy and was admitted at term with a blood pressure of 145/90 mm Hg. There were no further details except that the cervix failed to dilate after induction of labour, and that she was delivered by Caesarean section. She was discharged home on the 10th day, but died at home about a week later. An autopsy revealed a subarachnoid haemorrhage and an endocervical carcinoma. Although it was considered that the death was due to a cerebral aneurysm no identifiable source of vessel rupture was found.

b. *Cerebral infarction*

One woman had a postpartum carotid thrombosis with an extensive infarct of the right side of the brain. She developed symptoms on the ninth postpartum day. Her level of consciousness gradually deteriorated and she died several days later.

c. *Epilepsy*

There were only three deaths from epilepsy in this triennium as compared with seven in the 1982–84 report for England and Wales.

The first case is of a primipara, who had a history over many years of temporal lobe epilepsy for which she had been treated with anti-convulsants. When she became pregnant she had been off standard treatment and on a herbal medicine for some years, despite having several minor convulsions a day. She was not put on treatment by her general practitioner when she booked for shared care in this pregnancy. She continued to have convulsions but no attempt was made to treat her. At 32 weeks gestation she had a convulsion and she was found dead the following morning. Autopsy showed death was due to hypoxia which had probably occurred during a convulsion.

In the second case a primipara known to be an epileptic had a convulsion in bed at 15 weeks of pregnancy. At autopsy the blood pheno-barbitone level was found to be 0.4mg/100ml, which is well below the therapeutic level.

In the third case a young parous woman, known to be epileptic since childhood, was seen by her general practitioner in early pregnancy and was referred for hospital care and delivery. She was prescribed sodium valproate and carbamezapine in medical outpatients because her epilepsy was so poorly controlled.

Compliance with treatment was doubtful, but there is also no evidence that her therapy was monitored during pregnancy. At 33 weeks gestation she was found dead in her bathroom. A coroner's autopsy suggested that death was likely to have been due to an epileptic convulsion. Blood taken 36 hours after death suggested that the levels of anticonvulsants were sub-therapeutic although the significance of such measurements made so long after death is doubtful.

Substandard care

In all three women substandard care in the form of inadequate anti-convulsant therapy was implicated. In one case the general practitioner failed to recognise the need to insist on a woman restarting treatment because she was pregnant. In the second, the patient herself was responsible for failure to take prescribed treatment, and in the third a physician failed to recognise the importance in a known epileptic of determining appropriate anticonvulsant therapy by monitoring blood levels at regular intervals.

The message in the last report, and this one, is clear. Death in pregnancy amongst epileptics can be eliminated if both pregnant epileptics and their doctors are aware of the importance of maintaining treatment at all times in pregnancy and that the doses of anticonvulsant drugs necessary to maintain blood levels within the therapeutic range increase as pregnancy advances.

vii. **Disease of the circulatory system**

a. *Aneurysms*

The 1982–84 report for England and Wales identified a relationship between pregnancy and degenerative diseases of certain arteries. Excluding deaths from cerebral aneurysms there were 33 deaths in the 15 years from 1970–1984 inclusive, 19 of which were due to aortic aneurysms and 10 were due to splenic artery aneurysms. The situation is similar for the United Kingdom in 1985–87 when there were four deaths from aortic aneurysms and three deaths from splenic artery aneurysms.

Dissecting aortic aneurysms

In two of the four cases of aortic aneurysm there were conditions known to be associated with vascular defects in the aorta predisposing to the information of an aneurysm. In one case it was Marfan's syndrome and in the other multiple neurofibromatosis (von Recklinghausen's disease). However, in the latter case the woman also had a hypertensive disorder and her death has been counted as a Direct death in Chapter 2. There were, therefore, three Indirect deaths.

> The first, a parous woman with Marfan's syndrome, had acute chest pain at home, was admitted to the Casualty Department and collapsed shortly after her arrival there. Resuscitative measures were carried out to no avail and a postmortem Caesarean section was carried out. The baby, although born in poor condition, survived and is alive and well. The autopsy showed a horizontal tear in the aorta one cm above the right coronary artery and a dissecting aneurysm extending to just below the renal arteries, where there was a re-entry tear. The dissecting aneurysm had extended proximally and ruptured into the pericardial cavity giving rise to a haemopericardium.

> The second, a perfectly fit young woman, had an uneventful first pregnancy until she suddenly collapsed with chest pain near term. Cardiac arrest occurred and resuscitation failed. Autopsy revealed a dissecting aneurysm of the descending thoracic aorta. The tear partly involved the intrapericardial portion of the aorta and there was haemorrhagic dissection of the media down to both common iliac arteries, with a re-entry point in the left common iliac artery.

> The third woman had an uncomplicated first pregnancy and low forceps delivery and died suddenly due to an unsuspected aortic aneurysm. Autopsy revealed a haemopericardium resulting from a dissecting aneurysm involving the arch of the aorta.

There was no evidence of substandard care in these three Indirect deaths from dissecting aortic aneurysms.

ii. *Splenic artery aneurysms*

There were three deaths due to rupture of splenic artery aneurysms.

> The first death occurred in a young woman, who was admitted in her

first pregnancy at 34 weeks gestation with a suspected left sided urinary tract infection. Later that day she collapsed and died despite all resuscitative measures. Autopsy revealed a gross haemoperitoneum with rupture of a multisaccular aneurysm of the splenic artery. This was considered to be congenital in origin.

The second woman an apparently fit primigravida, had an uneventful first pregnancy, and was admitted at term in labour. After one hour in the second stage she collapsed at the height of a contraction, becoming cyanosed and hypotensive. An immediate forceps delivery was carried out. Resuscitation commenced, but it was unsuccessful. Autopsy revealed 2.5 1 of blood in the peritoneal cavity arising from a ruptured splenic artery aneurysm five cm from the splenic hilum.

The third death was in a fit primigravida who was admitted as an emergency with intra-abdominal bleeding at 21 week's gestation. Laparotomy revealed a massive splenic artery aneurysm which was ligated proximal and distal to the aneurysm. However bleeding continued and a very detailed autopsy revealed that the death of the patient was due to continued bleeding from the short gastric arteries.

There was no evidence of substandard care in any of the three deaths from splenic artery aneurysm, but it is of interest that all three women were pregnant for the first time.

Hereditary haemorrhagic telangiectasia

One young woman, with a history of hereditary telangiectasis, had the diagnosis made during her first pregnancy when it was thought she had a pulmonary embolus causing a haemoptysis. A chest X-ray revealed an arterio-venous malformation of the right lung. When in mid-pregnancy for the second time she had a painless haemoptysis from which she made a good recovery and was allowed home. A week later she had a further haemoptysis. Her condition deteriorated and she died. Autopsy confirmed a localised abnormality of the blood vessels in the right lung from which the bleeding had occurred. An incidental finding was a large vascular malformation in the brain. Although this woman could have died at any time because of the vascular abnormality, the death is considered to be an Indirect one because of the exacerbation of symptoms from the underlying abnormalities in both pregnancies.

Retroperitoneal haemorrhage

An elderly parous woman had three hospital admissions because of vomiting and loin pain with a diagnosis of renal colic which settled with analgesics. In her final admission she had several episodes of pain over a period of 24 hours and a Caesarean section at 33 weeks gestation was performed for suspected placental abruption. The Caesarean section was carried out without difficulty, but there was no evidence of abruption. A large left sided retroperitoneal haemorrhage was noted involving the left kidney and base of the broad ligament. During an unsuccessful attempt to establish the source of bleeding the patient had a cardiac arrest due to hypovolaemia. A meticulous autopsy suggested that the bleeding had arisen from an aneurysm of the renal vascular pedicle, but the precise site was not identified.

viii. Diseases of the respiratory system

Asthma

There was one Indirect death related to asthma. A further four due to asthma were classified as Fortuitous deaths.

This young woman died at home when 30 weeks pregnant in her first pregnancy from inhalation of vomit during an asthmatic attack.

ix. Diseases of the digestive system

Intestinal obstruction

An elderly parous woman, who suffered from external ophthalmoplegia associated with complete heart block, had a pacemaker in situ. She had a Caesarean section under epidural anaesthesia. Postoperatively she developed intestinal obstruction for which prolonged conservative measures were partially successful. It was planned for her to have a laparotomy, but her condition had deteriorated so much that she was unfit for operation. She had aspiration pneumonia, confirmed by chest X-ray, from which she died. Permission for autopsy was refused.

There was another death from intestinal obstruction after an ectopic pregnancy, which has been counted and described in Chapter 6.

x. Diseases of the genitourinary system

There were two Indirect deaths due to acute pyelonephritis and one Direct death, already discussed in Chapter 4, of a woman who had chronic glomerulonephritis and died from pulmonary embolism.

The first lady was admitted, severely ill, as an emergency with an incomplete, first trimester, abortion. There was evidence of septicaemia and DIC. The right kidney was tender and enlarged. An evacuation of the uterus under antibiotic cover was carried out within four hours of her admission, but she died within 24 hours of admission to hospital. Blood cultures taken during life revealed *Klebsiella* septicaemia. An inadequate autopsy revealed the right kidney to be enlarged and full of pus.

A parous woman was known to have had thrombocytopenic purpura in her previous pregnancies but did not book with her general practitioner until the twenty fifth week of pregnancy. She had an acute pyelonephritis at 27 weeks gestation treated by her general practitioner, but required admission two days later because of an antepartum haemorrhage. Later that day in the presence of septicaemia the membranes ruptured spontaneously and Caesarean section was performed because of fetal tachycardia. Despite antibiotic therapy she died a few days later. Autopsy confirmed the diagnosis of acute glomerular pyelonephritis.

The failure of this woman to book early with her general practitioner, particularly in view of her past history, resulted in her receiving substandard care.

xi. Diseases of the musculoskeletal system and connective tissues

a. *Still's disease*

A woman with Still's disease died from eclampsia and has been counted in Chapter 2.

b. *Kyphoscoliosis*

A woman with kyphoscoliosis died as the result of air embolism and has been described in Chapter 10.

xii. Sudden unnatural deaths

These included seven coroner's and two procurator fiscal's cases. Six deaths were considered to be suicide, one accidental, one misadventure and in one there was an open verdict. There were also four Late deaths which have been counted in Chapter 15.

a. *Suicide*

There were six deaths from suicide; five women had a history of psychiatric problems or developed puerperal psychosis, and there was one woman for whom these details were not available.

One highly parous woman, who had a puerperal psychosis, poured turpentine over herself and set it alight 17 days after delivery. She died the same evening.

Another young parous woman, with a previous placental abruption associated with a stillbirth, had received psychiatric treatment. She had already attempted suicide in her second pregnancy. Twenty-four hours prior to admission for a planned induction of labour because of her obstetric history, she committed suicide by carbon monoxide poisoning from car exhaust.

A young woman had a puerperal depression after a normal delivery at term of her first child and was under psychiatric care. Although she appeared to improve on medication, she was admitted via the Casualty department because of an overdose of paracetamol tablets. She was again discharged on treatment, but committed suicide by jumping out of a building.

A known drug addict, a parous woman, had a history of manic depression and was subject to mood swings. She had a spontaneous abortion and evacuation of the uterus under general anaesthesia. She died from an overdose of temazepam seven days later.

A young parous woman who had been treated by a child psychologist when aged 13–14 years, had many social problems. Thirty three days after delivery she was seen at home because of postnatal depression.

She was prescribed Prothiaden (dothiepin hydrochloride). The same evening she took all the tablets dispensed. No details of an autopsy were available.

The details for one young primigravida are minimal. She died of an overdose of theophylline which caused an acute cardio-respiratory arrest 27 days after delivery.

Comment

The history of previous psychiatric illness or disorders should alert all those involved in the care of women during and following pregnancy. Careful control of all medication prescribed is necessary.

Open verdict

One parous woman whose age was assumed to be about 40 years, had a 20 year history of depression with many episodes of manic and psychotic behaviour. She embarked on a pregnancy against medical advice and she required prolonged inpatient care in a psychiatric hospital. An elective Caesarean section was carried out at term and after a week she was transferred back to the psychiatric hospital from which she was discharged.

Thirty days after delivery she was found dead in the bath at home. Autopsy confirmed that death was due to drowning and suffocation from a plastic bag. Blood analysis also indicated excessive alcohol consumption.

Misadventure

A young parous woman who had an uneventful pregnancy and delivery at term, was discharged home after two days. She was found dead in the bath 11 days later. Autopsy revealed that she had drowned but had excessively high levels of alcohol. Although there was no evidence of depression or alcoholism and she was known to be only an occasional drinker, she had consumed a whole bottle of rum prior to taking a bath. The immediate cause of death was drowning.

Accidental death

A young woman, who sustained 40% burns in a house fire at 32 weeks gestation, was treated in a Regional burns unit. She died four days after admission from pulmonary oedema as a consequence of inhalation of smoke. It is possible that ritodrine, which was given to prevent the onset of labour, may have been a contributory factor.

Comment

Pregnancy, particularly in the latter stages, appears to have an adverse effect upon survival from burns of a pregnant female compared with a non-pregnant female of similar age and with a similar size of burn; and the chance of a live birth in a burned pregnant woman is worse than in the absence of burns. Reports on burns in pregnancy in the world literature are relatively scarce. It emerges from these studies that 40%

burns and a gestation of 32 weeks are each a watershed in their own right. Matthews advises that spontaneous labour should be suppressed in patients with burns up to 40% in the second and third trimester, the object being to improve the chance of fetal survival without worsening maternal prognosis[1]. Deitch et al believe that pharmacological inhibition of labour should be undertaken if the gestational age is between 24 and 32 weeks[2]. They point out, however, that the use of such agents as ritodrine in a woman with burns is not without risk and cite myocardial ischaemia and pulmonary oedema as possible side effects. Pulmonary oedema can occur in any extensively burned patient as a result of cardiovascular changes consequent upon fluid shifts that characterise the burn injury. The risk of pulmonary oedema is usually greatest at about 72 hours post-burn and is enhanced by lung damage due to smoke inhalation; it is often preceded by impairment of renal function[3].

Since the particular patient mentioned above had good renal function it should have substantially reduced her chance of developing pulmonary oedema 80 hours post-burn. Even though it is quite possible to explain the occurrence of pulmonary oedema in this woman without implicating ritodrine, it is acknowledged that it may have been a contributory factor.

The medical literature would, nevertheless, indicate that it is appropriate to use ritodrine to improve the chance of fetal survival between 24 and 32 weeks gestation.

References

1. Matthews R N. Obstetric implications of burns in pregnancy. Brit J Obs and Gyn 1982; *89*: 603–9.
2. Deitch, E A, Rightmire, J A. Clothier J, Blass N. Management of burns in pregnant women. Surg. Gyn and Obstet 1985; *161* (1): 1–4.
3. Amy B W, McManus W F, Goodwin C W, Mason A junior, Pruitt B A junior. Thermal injury in the pregnant patient. Surg. Gyn and Obstet 1985; *161* (3): 209–12.

CHAPTER 13

Caesarean section

Summary

There were 76 deaths following Caesarean section during the triennium and a further three where Caesarean section was carried out postmortem. Of these, 50 were Direct deaths, 22 Indirect deaths and four Fortuitous deaths. Care was judged to be substandard in 29 of the 50 Direct deaths and in five of the 22 Indirect deaths. In 23 cases there were substandard factors directly relating to the Caesarean section and associated aftercare.

In 11 cases Caesarean section was performed on mothers close to death and receiving cardiopulmonary support (perimortem cases). These sections, together with the three postmortem Caesarean sections, were primarily for fetal rescue but perinatal mortality was high (6 out of 14) and one survivor has spastic quadriplegia. Thus, excluding the peri- and postmortem sections, there were 46 Direct, 16 Indirect and three Fortuitous deaths in which delivery was by Caesarean section.

Caesarean section

During the years 1985–87 there were 76 deaths of women following delivery by Caesarean section (Table 13.1). Three postmortem Caesarean sections have been excluded from all the Tables. The 11 perimortem Caesarean sections have been included in the totals to permit comparison with previous triennia, and are indicated in parentheses.

Table 13.1 *Deaths connected with Caesarean section*, England and Wales 1970–87, compared with United Kingdom 1985–87.*

	Triennium	Total maternal deaths	Direct deaths	Indirect deaths	Fortuitous deaths	'Associated'** deaths
England & Wales	1970–72	102	81	—	—	21
	1973–75	77	60	—	—	17
	1976–78	80	61	14	5	—
	1979–81	87	59	25	3	—
	1982–84	69	44	20	5	—
	1985–87	64 (9)†	42 (3)†	19 (5)†	3 (1)†	
United Kingdom	1985–87	76 (11)†	50 (4)†	22 (6)†	4 (1)†	—

* Postmortem Caesarean sections excluded from all triennia.
** Associated deaths subdivided into Indirect and Fortuitous since 1976.
† Numbers in parentheses are the perimortem Caesarean sections in 1985–87.

The number of deaths in England and Wales associated with Caesarean section has continued to fall (Table 13.2). It is unfortunate that no data are

Table 13.2 Estimated number of Caesarean sections performed, and estimated fatality rate* per thousand Caesarean sections within 42 days in NHS hospitals in England and Wales for each triennium, England and Wales 1970–87, compared with United Kingdom 1985–87.

	Total maternities in NHS hospitals	Estimated number of Caesarean sections	Percentage of maternities by Caesarean section in NHS hospitals	Deaths after† Caesarean sections (Direct maternal and 'Associated' deaths from enquiry series)	Estimated fatality rate per thousand Caesarean sections
England & Wales 1970–72	2,000,612	103,310	5.2	102	0.99
1973–75	1,799,980	101,410	5.6	77	0.76
1976–78	1,689,670	120,570	7.1	80	0.66
1979–81	1,876,570	167,020	8.9	87	0.52
1982–84	1,840,970	185,820	10.1	69	0.37
1985–87	1,987,914**	N/A	N/A	64 (9)‡	N/A
United Kingdom 1985–87	2,231,797**	N/A	N/A	76 (11)‡	N/A

* Fatality rate for all deaths after Caesarean section, Direct and 'Associated' (after 1976 Indirect and Fortuitous)

** Total maternities in NHS Hospitals and elsewhere.

† Postmortem Caesarean sections excluded in all triennia.

‡ Numbers in parentheses are the perimortem Caesarean sections in 1985–87.

The collection of Hospital In-patient Statistics ended after 1985, to be replaced from 1987 onwards by new hospital episode statistics. Unfortunately at the time of writing these new data are not available, there are therefore no data about the number of Caesarean sections performed.

Table 13.3 Number of Direct maternal deaths within 42 days of Caesarean section,* England & Wales 1970–87, compared with United Kingdom, 1985–87.

	All Direct deaths	Direct deaths following Caesarean sections	Percentage of all Direct deaths	Caesarean section rate (%)	Estimated fatality rate/1,000 Caesarean sections
England & Wales 1970–72	343	81	24	5.16	0.78
1973–75	227	60	26	5.63	0.59
1976–78	217	61	28	7.14†	0.51
1979–81	178**	59	33	8.9†	0.35
1982–84	138	44	32	10.09	0.24
1985–87	121	42 (3)‡	35 (3)‡	N/A	N/A
United Kingdom 1985–87	139	50 (4)‡	36 (3)‡	N/A	N/A

* Postmortem Caesarean sections excluded in all triennia.

** Includes two other Direct deaths omitted from 1979–81 Report

† Revised figures to those previously published; corrected for error in calculation of total maternities in NHS hospitals.

‡ Numbers and percentages in parentheses are the perimortem Caesarean sections in 1985–87. (See text for definition of perimortem Caesarean section).

available on the numbers of Caesarean sections performed in NHS hospitals in England in this triennium and therefore there is no denominator for estimating the fatality rate. In England, Wales and Scotland the Caesarean section rate rose steadily during the previous five triennia. Data from Scotland and Wales show a continued rise in Caesarean section rate.

There has also been a slight fall in the number of Direct deaths following Caesarean section in England and Wales (Table 13.3) but they constitute a steadily increasing proportion of all Direct deaths (35% in 1985–87 compared with 24% in 1970–72).

Indications for Caesarean section in Direct maternal deaths

The principal indications for Caesarean section are shown in Table 13.4.

Table 13.4 *Indications for Caesarean sections* in Direct maternal deaths, United Kingdom 1985–87*

	Elective CS	Planned Emergency CS	Unplanned Emergency CS	Total
Hypertensive disorders	0	8	7	15
Fetal distress ± protracted labour	1	6	2	9
Protracted labour	0	5	0	5
Antepartum haemorrhage	0	1	3	4
Previous Caesarean section	3	1	0	4
Other obstetric conditions	0	2	2	4
Other maternal conditions	2	2	1	5
	6	25	15	46

* Perimortem Caesarean sections excluded

An unplanned emergency Caesarean section is defined as one where the need for operation overrides strict adherence to normal preparatory measures, such as a fasting period. This includes cases in which elective Caesarean section had been planned but was pre-empted by clinical events. A planned emergency section is one in which appropriate preparatory care has been followed, that is for patients in labour, that they have fasted, been given antacids and been fully assessed.

Immediate causes of death following Caesarean section

The attributed causes of death following Caesarean section are shown in Table 13.5 with comparisons for previous triennia for England and Wales.

The major causes of death remain the same, with hypertensive disorders now being the main hazard. Four of the hypertensive deaths were due to intracranial haemorrhage and four to adult respiratory distress syndrome (ARDS). There was a substantial fall in the deaths directly attributed to anaesthesia and this is further commented on in Chapter 9.

Table 13.5 *The number and the percentage in parentheses of all deaths after Caesarean section+ classified according to immediate cause of death, England & Wales 1970–87*** compared with United Kingdom, 1985–87*

		Haemorrhage	Pulmonary embolus	Sepsis	Hypertensive disease	Anaesthesia	Other Direct causes	Indirect and fortuitous*	Total
England & Wales	1970–72	8 (8)	15 (15)	15 (15)	13 (13)	22 (22)	8 (8)	21 (21)	102
	1973–75	8 (10)	6 (8)	8 (10)	12 (16)	17 (22)	9 (12)	17 (22)	77
	1976–78	8 (10)	9 (11)	8 (10)	12 (15)	18 (22)	6 (8)	19 (24)	80
	1979–81	7 (8)	7 (8)	4 (5)	13 (15)	19 (22)	9 (10)	28 (32)	87
	1982–84	4 (6)	12 (17)	1 (1)	10 (14)	8 (12)	9 (13)	25 (36)	69
	1985–87	5 (8)	4 (6)	2 (3)	14 (22)	3 (5)	14 (22)	22 (34)	64†
United Kingdom	1985–87	5 (7)	9 (12)**	2 (3)	14 (18)	4 (5)	16 (21)	26 (34)	76†

† Perimortem Caesarean sections are included (see text for definition).
* Associated deaths subdivided in Indirect and Fortuitous deaths since 1976.
** Includes one death from arterial thrombosis.
*** Postmortem Caesarean sections are excluded for all triennia.

Direct and Indirect deaths

A breakdown of the 62 Direct and Indirect deaths, excluding the perimortem Caesarean sections, is given in Table 13.6.

Table 13.6 *Direct and Indirect deaths* related to elective and emergency procedures.*

	Deaths		
	Direct	Indirect	Total
Elective	6	2	8
Planned emergency	25	8	33
Unplanned emergency	15	6	21
Total	46	16	62

* Perimortem Caesarean sections excluded.

Elective Caesarean sections

Five of the eight elective sections were repeat operations. Four of these were Direct deaths due to air embolism, amniotic fluid embolism, retroperitoneal haemorrhage and anaesthetic complications. Only in the last case, described in Chapter 9, was substandard care implicated. The fifth repeat operation was in a patient with primary pulmonary hypertension and was an Indirect cardiac death. The other three elective sections were as follows:–

A young multigravida had an elective section for antenatal fetal distress. The procedure and postpartum period were uneventful but she died from a pulmonary embolism 35 days postpartum.

A primigravida with aortic valve disease collapsed during administration of epidural analgesia and the details are discussed in Chapter 9.

A young primigravida suffered from diabetes and had an elective section for antenatal fetal distress. She died from bronchopneumonia eight days postpartum.

Indirect and Fortuitous deaths

There were 23 Indirect deaths and four Fortuitous deaths, as detailed in Table 13.7. In six cases Caesarean section was performed whilst patients were having terminal cardiopulmonary resuscitation (perimortem).

Fortuitous deaths

There were four Fortuitous deaths. In three cases the Caesarean section was irrelevant and death in the puerperium was due to carcinoma of the rectum, astrocytoma and carcinoma of the breast respectively. In the fourth case Caesarean section was undertaken after brain death in a patient with astrocytoma. In no case was there evidence of substandard care.

Classification and cause of death	Number
Indirect deaths	
Septicaemia	1
Varicella pneumonia	1
Bronchopneumonia	1
Sickle cell haemoglobinopathy	1
Primary pulmonary hypertension	1
Infective endocarditis	1
Ischaemic heart disease	2
Retroperitoneal haematoma	1
Carcinomatosis	1
Phaeochromocytoma	1
Intestinal obstruction	1
Cerebral haemorrhage	3
Sudden unexpected death	1
Peri and Post-mortem Caesarean section in Indirect deaths	
Mycobacterium infection	1
Primary pulmonary hypertension	1
Ruptured aortic aneurysm	1
Cerebral haemorrhage	4
Fortuitous deaths	
Carcinoma of rectum	1
Carcinoma of breast	1
Cerebral tumour	1
Perimortem Caesarean section in Fortuitous deaths	
Cerebral tumour	1

Peri- and postmortem Caesarean sections

There were fourteen peri- and postmortem Caesarean sections performed.

Perimortem Caesarean sections

The term perimortem has been used for those eleven cases where the patient was moribund or in extremis, was on cardiopulmonary resuscitation prior to the Caesarean section and showed no signs of recovery thereafter. Four of these were Direct obstetric deaths, six were Indirect deaths and one was Fortuitous.

Postmortem Caesarean section

In these three cases the patient was dead on arrival at hospital and no attempts at resuscitation were made. Two of the three postmortem cases were Direct deaths and one Indirect. All were believed to have died suddenly at least 30 minutes before admission and all had Caesarean sections undertaken in the Accident and Emergency Department. Two babies were stillborn. The third had an Apgar score of two at one minute but made a rapid and good recovery. There was no obvious neurological deficit at the time of the child's discharge from hospital.

Perimortem Caesarean section

In the eleven patients sectioned whilst having cardiopulmonary resuscitation the operation was primarily carried out for fetal rescue but occasionally also as an aid to maternal management.

Four women collapsed at home, two with subarachnoid haemorrhage, one with pulmonary embolism and one with a ruptured aortic aneurysm. Gestational age was over 34 weeks in all cases.

All the babies survived, but one, in which the interval from collapse to delivery was approximately 40 minutes, has spastic quadriplegia.

> One patient died in the cardiac operating theatre during thoracotomy for constrictive pericarditis. Caesarean section was done by the cardiac surgeon. The baby, of 28 weeks gestation, weighed 1.25kg and died after 12 hours from intracranial haemorrhage.

> A patient in an intensive care unit (ICU) with a brain tumour was considered to have brain death at 30 weeks gestation, and 12 hours later a Caesarean section was carried out. The infant, weighing 1.52kg, survived.

Five patients collapsed whilst in the Delivery Unit, two from amniotic fluid embolism, one from pulmonary hypertension, one from subarachnoid haemorrhage and one with unexplained sudden collapse in labour. Cardiopulmonary resuscitation was established promptly in all cases. The interval from collapse to Caesarean section ranged from 30 to 60 minutes. Two of the babies were stillborn (both associated with amniotic fluid embolism — the interval to delivery being 40 minutes and 60 minutes respectively). One baby died early in the neonatal period as a result of asphyxia (unexplained sudden maternal collapse — interval to delivery 30 minutes). The other two babies survived; the time interval was not recorded in either case.

In this series of perimortem Caesarean sections there were eight surviving infants, but one baby had spastic quadriplegia. The two neonatal deaths and the quadriplegic baby were all born to mothers who were on life support apparatus. In addition two of the three infants delivered by post-mortem Caesarean section were stillborn.

Comment

In situations where peri- and postmortem sections may be undertaken clear policies must be established and appropriate facilities provided as far as possible.

At least four of the surviving babies in this triennium were in poor condition at birth and required resuscitation, but in only one of these is there a record of a paediatrician being on site. If effective cardiopulmonary resuscitation has been established for the mother a less hasty approach to Caesarean section for fetal rescue might be appropriate so that the services of a neonatologist and appropriate equipment could be obtained either in the delivery unit or the ICU.

Substandard care

In 23 cases there was substandard care of direct relevance to the Caesarean section and postoperative management.

Availability of facilities

In eight cases, all delivered in consultant units, there was specific mention of the absence of intensive care facilities on the site, which may have been a contributory factor. In seven of these cases the section was for obstetric indications (failed induction; prolapsed cord; placental abruption, two cases; failed forceps; fetal distress, two cases). In the eighth case the Caesarean section was in a patient with subarachnoid haemorrhage. In addition there were two cases in which it was considered that delivery should have been arranged in the cardiothoracic unit. The report of the Maternity Services Advisory Committee (Maternity Care in Action Part 2[1]) emphasised the need to integrate obstetric services with district general hospitals. The above cases illustrate the relevance and importance of this recommendation in that five Caesarean sections were for conventional obstetric indications which would be standard in any consultant unit but in which unexpected complications developed. Also, units isolated from acute district general hospital sites often lack not only an ICU but also skilled staff able to cope with acute catastrophes and adequate readily available supplies of blood.

Inappropriate delegation

In nine cases there appeared to be inappropriate delegation of Caesarean section and associated care to junior staff. In four cases the operator was a locum or acting registrar and in some cases problems were compounded by having an inexperienced anaesthetist, a combination which can readily lead to inappropriate management decisions when major problems arise.

Six of the nine patients had eclampsia or severe pre-eclampsia. For management of such cases an adequate experienced team is necessary and junior staff should not be expected to cope with peri- and intraoperative management as well as performing the surgery.

Inadequate consultation

In at least four cases there was clearly failure of consultation and co-ordination with other professional colleagues which might have aided in the management of complications following Caesarean section.

Other examples of substandard care not directly related to Caesarean section are mentioned in the appropriate chapters.

Reference

1. Munro A. Maternity Care in Action Part II Care During Childbirth (Intrapartum care): second report of the Maternity Services Advisory Committee to the Secretaries to State for Social Services and Wales. London: HMSO 1984. Chairman: Mrs Alison Munro.

CHAPTER 14

Fortuitous deaths

Fortuitous deaths are those deaths due to non-obstetric causes which happen coincidentally in pregnancy or the puerperium. By international definition such deaths are not considered as part of maternal mortality. These deaths are listed in Table 15.1

In 1985–87 there were 26 Fortuitous deaths reported to the enquiry.

Table 14.1 *Fortuitous deaths*

Cause of death	Number
Infectious disease	
Viral hepatitis B	1
Neoplastic disease	
Carcinoma of stomach	1
Carcinoma of rectum	1
Malignant melanoma	1
Carcinoma of breast	1
Cerebral astrocytoma	3
Non-Hodgkin's lymphoma	1
Neurolemmoma	1
Blood disease	
Acute monoblastic leukaemia	2
Myelomonocytic leukaemia	1
Disease of nervous system	
Viral meningitis	1
Streptococcal meningitis	1
Disease of circulatory system	
Endocarditis	1
Coronary atheroma	1
Disease of respiratory system	
Asthma	4
Sudden unnatural deaths	
Accident	
Road traffic accident, multiple injuries	4
Open verdict	
House fire	1
Total	26

CHAPTER 15

Late deaths

Deaths in women more than 42 days, but less than one year after pregnancy or delivery are defined as Late deaths.

In 1985–87 only 16 Late deaths were reported to the United Kingdom Enquiry. This compared with 73 Late deaths for England and Wales alone in 1982–84. This fall was due to a decision taken by the assessors for England and Wales in 1984, that deaths over 42 days would be excluded from the 1985–87 Report, in line with the International Definition of Maternal Deaths. It was then agreed that considerable unnecessary work was being undertaken in collecting information for these Late deaths, many of which were also considered to be Fortuitous, that is unrelated to pregnancy and delivery.

However, it was soon realised that strict adherence to this new rule was resulting in the exclusion of a few deaths which were almost certainly related to pregnancy. Therefore some Late deaths which were considered by the Regional Assessors to be of interest to the enquiry were reported, and have been included. For the next triennium 1988–90, it was recommended that all deaths up to six months after pregnancy or delivery should be reported, and that District Medical Officers (or Directors of Public Health) should discuss any cases dying between six months and one year with the English Regional or Welsh assessors, who would advise whether or not they should be reported to the enquiry.

Scotland and Northern Ireland have continued to collect cases up to one year after pregnancy or delivery.

Direct maternal deaths

Six of the Late deaths were considered to be Direct maternal deaths, despite the time which had elapsed since delivery.

One death was due to recurrent pulmonary thromboembolism. A parous woman had a normal pregnancy and delivery and was well on discharge from hospital. She saw her general practitioner early in the puerperium with swelling of the legs which improved with treatment. She was fitted with an intra-uterine device and so did not take a contraceptive pill. For some weeks before her death, more than five months after delivery, she was breathless, but did not consult her doctor. She then collapsed at home and died the same day in hospital. At autopsy both main pulmonary arteries and some smaller arteries were blocked with fresh thrombus. There were also older thrombi of at least four weeks duration, and she had bilateral pleural effusions.

These findings suggested recurrent small pulmonary emboli causing pulmonary haemorrhage without infarction and ultimately leading to right heart failure.

> A young primigravida was admitted in labour at term. She had epidural analgesia, and was treated with antibiotics for a pyrexia starting before delivery. She required an emergency Caesarean section for fetal distress. Postoperatively she developed disseminated intravascular coagulation (DIC) and was treated the following day by subtotal hysterectomy for continuing vaginal bleeding. She became oliguric, jaundiced and also had respiratory problems. Despite expert treatment in an intensive care unit (ICU) which included haemodialysis for renal failure and treatment for recurrent septicaemia, she died three months postpartum. Autopsy confirmed hepato-renal failure and septicaemia, considered to have originated from genital tract sepsis.

Two women died from choriocarcinoma.

> The first patient, a parous woman, was admitted to hospital before term, with chest pain and haemoptysis. Communication difficulties caused problems throughout the case, both with obtaining her medical history and keeping in touch with her on discharge. She was reviewed by a chest physician who decided that she did not have a recurrence of a previous tuberculous infection. When she was in early labour, a controlled ARM was performed because of excess fluid and two litres were removed. Later at Caesarean section, performed for fetal bradycardia, a large, hydropic, stillborn baby was delivered. Six days later a laparotomy was performed because sepsis was suspected of causing abdominal distension but only ascites was found. She was discharged home about four weeks postpartum. A week later she attended hospital because of vaginal bleeding, and had a D and C two days later. After she had left hospital the curettings were reported as showing choriocarcinoma.

> There was difficulty and delay in contacting the patient, re-admitting her to hospital and then in trying to arrange her transfer to a specialist unit. A CT scan then showed cerebral metastases and chemotherapy was started, but she died two weeks later, over two months postpartum.

> The second patient, a primigravida, had a normal pregnancy and delivery. Her general practitioner performed her postnatal examination and later confirmed that she had had prolonged vaginal bleeding. From about two months after delivery she had intermittent episodes of nausea, visual disturbance and occasional headaches. Four months after delivery she was admitted to hospital with a 24-hour history of severe headache, nausea and vomiting. A CT scan on admission showed multiple cerebral metastases, and an X-ray examination multiple deposits in the lungs. A raised serum beta-hCG level confirmed the diagnosis of choriocarcinoma. She was transferred to a specialist unit and chemotherapy was started. However she had a respiratory arrest and died the following day. Autopsy confirmed multiple metastases form choriocarcinoma.

There was considered to have been substandard care in the delay in diagnosis and treatment of both these cases.

Two patients died as the result of anaesthetic complications at delivery, and have been described in Chapter 9.

Indirect and Fortuitous Late deaths.

There was eight Indirect maternal deaths and two Fortuitous deaths. They have been listed in Tables 15.1 and 15.2 respectively.

Table 15.1 *Late Indirect maternal deaths*

Cause of death	Number
Disease of circulatory system	
Cardiomyopathy	1
Intracerebral haemorrhage and subdural haemorrhage	1
Intracerebral haemorrhage	1
Other condition of the mother complicating pregnancy, childbirth or puerperium	
Unexplained death	1
Sudden unnatural death	
Suicide*	
Overdose	1
Hanging	2
*Misadventure**	
Hepatic failure due to drug reaction	1
Total	8

* All under treatment for puerperal depression

Table 15.2 *Late Fortuitous deaths*

Cause of death	Number
Neoplastic disease	
Carcinoma of breast	1
Sudden unnatural deaths	
Accidental	
Road Traffic Accident	1
Total	2

Table 15.3 *The interval in days between delivery or abortion and death in the Late cases United Kingdom 1985–87.*

Days between delivery or abortion and death	Direct deaths	Indirect deaths	Fortuitous deaths	Total
43–91	1	5	1	7
92–182	3	2	1	6
183–273	—	—	—	1
274–365	2	—	—	2
Total	6	8	2	16

Table 15.4 *The interval in days between delivery or abortion and death in the Late cases England and Wales 1976–87, and England and Wales 1985–87, and United Kingdom 1985–87.*

Days between delivery or abortion and death	1976–87 England and Wales				1985–87 E & W Total	1985–87 UK Total
	Direct	Indirect	Fortuitous	Total		
43–91	12	27	37	76	6	7
92–182	10	18	58	86	5	6
183–273	2	8	25	35	1	1
274–365	5	3	24	32	2	2
Total	29	56	144	229	14	16

Table 15.3 shows the interval in days between delivery or abortion and death for the three groups of Late cases in 1985–87. Table 15.4 shows the same information for England and Wales only for the four triennia since 1976, and the totals for 1985–87 for England and Wales separately and for the United Kingdom.

CHAPTER 16

Pathology

Summary

Of the 265 deaths reviewed in this report autopsies were performed on 215 (81%). In a further three cases examination was limited, in two to examination of the liver (one by needle biopsy) and in the third to examination of a kidney. Subjectively the autopsy reports were considered to be satisfactory in 155 (very good or good in 91 and adequate in 64) but unsatisfactory in 60. Histology was considered satisfactory in 113 and unsatisfactory or there was no report in 102.

The quality of the autopsy

Although in the last report the standard of autopsy following maternal death was considered to have improved, this report reveals that there is still a disturbing number of autopsies which are considered to be substandard.

Autopsies performed at the request of HM Coroners/Procurators Fiscal

There is a widespread belief that these autopsies merely require to establish a registrable cause of death. Beyond this, however, both coroners/procurators fiscal and pathologists have a duty of responsibility to provide as much information as possible about complex cases and a detailed autopsy report is required in all cases. When the coroner/procurator fiscal does not order an autopsy the clinicians should seek permission from the next of kin in the normal way. In this 1985–87 report the coroner/procurator fiscal did not order an autopsy to establish the nature of the heart disease in two cases of congenital heart disease, although one of the patients died on the operating table undergoing emergency cardiac surgery. Infective endocarditis could not be excluded. In another three cases the coroner authorised the removal of organs for transplantation but was not prepared to authorise an autopsy to examine the genital organs. Such reluctance is a serious limitation of the investigation of these deaths.

Pathologists performing autopsies for coroners/procurators fiscal frequently rely upon preprinted forms to record their observations. Such forms may permit little space for recording important details or weights of organs and the inadequacy of many reports was related to this imposed brevity. The worst example of an inadequate report consisted of seven short lines of comment without any description of the genital organs.

Hypertension

In deaths associated with hypertensive disorders of pregnancy, gross and microscopic examination of the uterus and placental bed, the placenta, kidneys, heart, liver and brain is essential. In this report, there were 27 deaths attributed to pregnancy-induced hypertension (pre-eclampsia or eclampsia). There was no autopsy in two of these and the autopsy was considered inadequate in seven. In one of the two cases without a full autopsy a kidney was removed for histological examination. In 12 of the cases there was no histology report (seven) or an inadequate histological examination (five). In an additional three cases without a histology report the Regional Pathology Assessor was able to obtain blocks/sections for examination and this formed the basis of the histological diagnosis. In three of the five cases with an inadequate histological report histology was limited to the kidney (one), liver and kidney (one) and lung (one); in the remaining two, one case had severely autolysed tissues unsuitable for detailed histology and the other had poor histological descriptions and little correlation with the gross findings. In most of the reports more emphasis was given to the changes of adult respiratory distress syndrome (ARDS) than to the uterine or renal changes.

Adult respiratory distress syndrome

The diagnosis of ARDS (shock lung) has been made more frequently in this than in previous reports. For example, in patients with hypertensive disorders of pregnancy (Chapter 2), ARDS ranked second (9/25) to intra-cerebral haemorrhage (11/25) as the immediate cause of death. This high frequency, not noted in previous Confidential Enquiries, may be due partly to its more frequent recognition by pathologists and partly to patients surviving longer, thus allowing time for the disease to become established.

ARDS may result from a wide variety of causes including septicaemia, shock, fluid overload, high concentration of inhaled oxygen, and inhaled gastric contents. It is regarded as a final common pathway of diffuse alveolar damage. Three phases are recognised, a pre-clinical phase, an early acute exudative phase and a later proliferative clinical phase. The first phase is seen mainly in experimental models and results in capillary leak due to damaged alveolar capillary endothelial cells and Type 1 pneumo-cytes (epithelial cells) caused by polymorphonuclear leucocytes. These cells cause damage either as a result of the release of lysosomal proteolytic enzymes or due to the generation of oxygen free-radicals which damage cell membranes. The second, or early acute exudative phase, develops in the first week following injury. As a result of capillary leakage there is oedema of the alveolar septa and into the alveolar lumen causing hypoxaemia. During this phase hyaline membranes form and line the alveolar septa. These membranes consist of necrotic cell debris, protein and fibrin. In the third, late phase, which develops after a further 1–2 weeks, there is proliferation of Type 2 pneumocytes and fibrosis mainly of the alveolar lumen. Diffuse pulmonary fibrosis develops in some survivors.

The exudative phase is that seen most commonly at autopsy. The lungs are heavy and plum coloured. Although fluid may exude from the cut surface it is more difficult to express than from oedematous lungs following heart failure or fluid overload, presumably because much of the oedema in

ARDS is in the interstitium rather than in the air spaces. There is commonly accompanying bronchopneumonia. Until the pathophysiology of ARDS is more clearly established it is important for pathologists to identify the disease at autopsy and to take sufficient histology to establish a diagnosis.

Antepartum and postpartum haemorrhage

There were 10 deaths due to antepartum or postpartum haemorrhage in one of which there was no autopsy. One of the autopsies was considered inadequate because the source of the fatal intraperitoneal haemorrhage was not identified. In five autopsies there was an inadequate histology report or none at all. Histological confirmation of the anatomical diagnosis is of particular importance in cases of obstetric haemorrhage, where it is critical in establishing evidence for the two main predisposing conditions of amniotic fluid embolism and disseminated intravascular coagulation (DIC). Any report on such a case which does not include a specific comment on this matter based on histological evidence must be seen as inadequate. Pathologists should also be aware of the importance of a full report on any previous hysterectomy specimen which may take on a particular significance in a retrospective analysis.

Thrombosis and thromboembolism

There were 30 deaths from pulmonary embolism, including one following an abortion counted in Chapter 6. Autopsies were performed on all but four of these cases but the histological report was inadequate or absent in 13. The site of the primary thrombosis was not identified in seven cases due to inadequate examination of the pelvic and leg veins. In one instance pulmonary infarction was described but the pulmonary vasculature was not mentioned in the report.

> The woman was known to have hereditary telangiectasia and had suffered from repeated epistaxes. At 36 weeks gestation she developed tingling in the arms and hands and telephoned her general practitioner. A short time later she was found lying lifeless on the floor, was taken to the neighbouring Accident and Emergency department and a post-mortem Caesarean section was performed. At autopsy the lungs were described as being infarcted. The cause of death was given as cardiac failure due to recurrent small calibre emboli originating in the pelvic veins, although these were not described in the report nor was there comment on the appearance of the pulmonary arteries.

It would be unusual for sudden death to occur, as in this case, from recurrent small pulmonary emboli, nor would pulmonary infarction be anticipated if death occurred suddenly after a massive pulmonary embolus. Although coded to pulmonary embolism, doubt must remain concerning the cause of death in this case.

> Another young woman who was a known epileptic, collapsed and died at 31 weeks gestation. At autopsy she was found to have a pulmonary embolus associated with thrombosis of the deep veins of the left calf. Examination of the heart revealed that it was dilated and, surprisingly,

there were changes interpreted as an antero-septal infarct of the left ventricle. However, histology, which was limited to the left ventricular myocardium, showed changes of chronic myocarditis.

A diagnosis of antero-septal myocardial infarction without coronary artery occlusion in a young woman should have alerted the pathologist to the possibility of myocarditis and appropriate samples of blood and myocardium should have been retained for microbiological examination. The cause of the myocarditis remains unknown. This case emphasises the need for blood to be retained for bacterial, viral and toxicological studies and for full histological examination of all organs, but especially the heart, in cases of sudden death.

Amniotic fluid embolism

A diagnosis of death due to amniotic fluid embolism requires positive evidence of amniotic fluid in the maternal circulation. All nine proven cases in this report, as in previous reports, required an autopsy with histological examination of the pulmonary vasculature to establish the diagnosis. In one case no amniotic fluid constituents could be found in the pulmonary vasculature but amniotic squames were found in the myometrial veins of the hysterectomy specimen removed eight days prior to death. This case emphasises the importance of examination of hysterectomy specimens in all cases of maternal death. It is fortunate that a meticulous examination of the hysterectomy specimen and a detailed autopsy were performed by an experienced histopathologist.

> The patient developed signs of amniotic fluid embolism during delivery and suffered severe postpartum haemorrhage necessitating hysterectomy. She was transferred to an intensive care unit (ICU) where she was maintained on ventilation for eight days before she died. At autopsy the lungs showed changes of ARDS but no amniotic fluid remnants were identified in the many blocks examined. It was concluded that the amniotic fluid had been cleared from the pulmonary vasculature during the interval of intensive therapy. If detailed examination of the hysterectomy specimen had not been performed the extensive permeation of the uterine veins by amniotic fluid would not have been detected.

In a further two cases death was attributed to uterine rupture although amniotic fluid embolism was also found at autopsy.

In nine more patients, three with placental abruption and six with postpartum haemorrhage, coagulation defects were diagnosed clinically. In one of the patients there was a previously undiagnosed Factor VIII deficiency. In none of the cases was amniotic fluid embolism confirmed.

Care must be taken in applying the criteria for diagnosing amniotic fluid embolism. The demonstration of amniotic squames in the maternal circulation allows a confident diagnosis but small quantities of lipid or mucin in alveolar capillaries in the absence of squames must be treated with caution. One such case was excluded because the baby was born with intact fetal membranes and the diagnosis of amniotic fluid embolism was made only on the presence of minimal quantities of alveolar lipid which could not be confirmed later. The use of immunohistological stains for cytokeratins is a useful adjunct for the detection of amniotic squames. Where amniotic fluid embolism is suspected, pulmonary arterial blood should be examined using a routine Romanowsky stained smear. This is a simple way to detect squames and the sensitivity may be increased by using the buffy coat in a centrifuged specimen.

Early pregnancy deaths (including abortions)

There were 16 deaths attributed to ectopic pregnancy. In one there was no autopsy and in four the autopsy report was considered inadequate due to the paucity of information provided. There was no histological report in nine and an inadequate histological report in one.

In one patient with a ruptured tubal pregnancy the preoperative haemoglobin concentration was 4.6g/dl. She was known to have sickle-cell trait. There was further severe blood loss during and following surgery. The patient developed severe pulmonary oedema and died. No organ weights were given in the autopsy report to assess the severity of the pulmonary oedema and there was no histology to assess whether the haemoglobinopathy had contributed to death.

A second case, a woman who had had a total colectomy and ileostomy for ulcerative colitis, was found to have an abdominal pregnancy with erosion of the small bowel by the placenta. She developed a *Cl. perfringens* septicaemia and DIC leading to death. Although the gross description of the autopsy was adequate and suggested ARDS no histology was taken to confirm this diagnosis or DIC.

Of the six deaths due to abortion there was no autopsy in one. The autopsy was considered inadequate in a further two and there was no histological report in three.

Genital tract sepsis

Previous recommendations about blood and organ culture are frequently not being observed. In the six Direct deaths due to genital tract sepsis in this report no culture was taken of the genital tract at autopsy in two and there was no histology report in two. As a result of inadequate microbiological and histological examination one further Direct death was reclassified as unexplained.

The patient had a Caesarean section performed for prolapsed cord. On the fourth postoperative day she developed signs of septicaemia, although cultures of blood, urine and lochia were negative. Her condition became worse and it was thought there was intraperitoneal bleeding. At laparotomy an abdominal wall haematoma was noted but there was no intraperitoneal bleeding. She developed features of DIC and died three days after laparotomy. The autopsy report was grossly inadequate with little description of the organs. No cultures were taken and there was no histology to confirm either DIC or infection. Although a confident diagnosis was given to the coroner of genital sepsis leading to gram negative septicaemia this diagnosis was quite unsubstantiated.

Three deaths, two Indirect and one sudden unexplained antepartum death, had been attributed to septicaemia following acute pyelonephritis. In none of these cases was the kidney cultured and in one case no histology was taken.

Genital tract trauma

Five of these six cases came to autopsy. In four there was a full anatomical description, with appropriate histology; in two of these, where a hysterectomy had been carried out prior to death, a full report on the separate surgical specimen was included.

In the fifth case, the autopsy report was no more than adequate. There was no description of the histological findings, although tissue for histology was apparently taken, nor of the previously resected uterus. In the sixth case, it was reported that autopsy permission was refused. This early postoperative maternal death should certainly have fallen within the coroner's jurisdiction.

Although it is sometimes difficult to define an 'anatomical' cause of death in instances of genital trauma with fatal haemorrhage, a full postmortem examination is still essential in every case. The pathologist should ascertain the presence and extent of injuries and of any concealed haemorrhage; should determine whether injuries identified at the time of a previous hysterectomy extend further than was clinically suspected at operation; and should seek evidence of amniotic fluid embolism and DIC as factors possibly contributing to death through haemorrhage. A detailed report on any separate hysterectomy specimen is essential in the assessment of such cases.

Other Direct deaths

There were 20 other Direct deaths of which 12 were unexplained. There was no autopsy in one of these and an inadequate autopsy in a further seven. In four there was no histological examination and in another four the histological examination was inadequate. Three of these unexplained deaths were attributed initially to septicaemia but there was no positive bacteriological culture during life and in two there was no culture taken at autopsy. In the third death there was no autopsy. The diagnosis of septicaemia was therefore not confirmed.

In another case death was attributed at autopsy to diabetic ketoacidosis although there was no past history of diabetes. At only one antenatal examination was glycosuria detected but there was no ketoacidosis. A post-prandial blood sugar was 6.4 mmol/l. The woman was later found dead in bed having vomited. The major air passages were described at autopsy as normal and patent without inhaled stomach contents. On review, the diagnosis of diabetic ketoacidosis was not considered to be substantiated.

Air embolism

The detection of air embolism at autopsy requires the pathologist to be aware of this possibility before the start of the autopsy. When air embolism is a possibility a chest x-ray is desirable before the autopsy commences. Similarly, before any major vein is opened, the pathologist must ensure that the inferior and superior vena cavae are inspected and the right atrium and right ventricle must be opened under water. In the three cases of air embolism in this report there is no indication that such a procedure was adopted.

Deaths associated with Anaesthesia

Eight deaths, including two Late deaths, were directly attributable to anaesthesia and in two of these there was no autopsy. In four cases the autopsy report was considered to be inadequate because of a poor anatomical description and in only two cases was the autopsy report adequate. There was no histology report in three cases and in one case it was confined to the lung. In three of the cases, the conclusion of the autopsy was that the patient had died of cerebral hypoxia but the description of the gross appearance of the brain was poor and there was no histological confirmation of the changes. These three cases of inadequate examination of the brain undertaken on the instructions of coroners/procurators fiscal are in striking contrast to other autopsies reviewed in the 1985–87 report, where cerebral pathology has been suspected and the brain has been submitted to a neuropathologist for examination. The standard of the latter examinations has been excellent, providing detailed information of great value.

Four deaths were associated with difficulty of tracheal intubation. One of these patients who was undergoing Caesarean section died on the operating table. In the autopsy report there was no description of the tracheal tube location. This failure draws attention to the necessity for the tracheal tube and all other lines and drains to be left in situ and for their position to be accurately recorded in the report.

One patient died following regurgitation and inhalation of stomach contents during induction of anaesthesia. The standard of both the autopsy and the histology was good and there was extensive histological examination of the lungs. The diagnosis of pneumonitis due to inhalation of stomach contents may be difficult in the presence of the changes of ARDS due to other causes. Multiple blocks of lung from all lobes should be examined to detect inhaled foreign material or peptic digestion.

Cardiac disease

There were 23 cardiac deaths of which one was considered Direct, and a further two in which cardiac disease contributed to death. Of the Indirect cardiac deaths there was no autopsy in three and the autopsy was considered inadequate in a further three. In one of the latter there was a poor, brief description of the organs which did not correlate with the histology. In the remaining two cases, both of pulmonary hypertension, no attempt was made to assess the severity of right ventricular hypertrophy.

In three cases there was no histology. In one of these cases there was an anatomical diagnosis of infective endocarditis and rheumatic mitral stenosis.

In the other two there was a diagnosis of ischaemic heart disease, one in an elderly postpartum diabetic woman and the other in a young woman with a 12 week gestation. Both showed coronary artery occlusion due to atheroma.

In three cases histology was considered inadequate. In one of these, a case of infective endocarditis, there was no histology of the heart. In a case of primary pulmonary hypertension, histology was limited to one block from the lung and in a case of myocardial ischaemia histology was not taken from the ischaemic area of the heart.

These cases illustrate the importance of a detailed anatomical examination of the heart, if necessary including the weights of the isolated left and right ventricles to assess hypertrophy. Histological and, if relevant, microbiological examination should also be undertaken. Histological examination should include other sites in the cardiovascular system if systemic vascular disease is suspected.

Other Indirect causes of maternal death

Aneurysms

In previous reports for England and Wales attention has been drawn to the increased prevalence of aneurysms in pregnancy. A careful search for the stigmata of Marfan's syndrome or for generalised vascular disease is required, including detailed histological examination of the aneurysm and other arteries. In this report 12 deaths were attributed to ruptured aneurysms and one to dissection of a coronary artery. In a further six cases, diagnosed as subarachnoid haemorrhage, the source of the bleeding was not identified. In three of these there was no autopsy and in a further case the autopsy was inadequate because there was no description of the cerebral arteries. Five of the 12 ruptured aneurysms occurred in vessels arising from the circle of Willis, three in the splenic artery and four in the aorta. There was no autopsy in three of these cases, all with subarachnoid haemorrhage from leaking cerebral aneurysms confirmed by computerised tomography. There was no postmortem histology in a further six cases. In one of these the splenic artery was examined histologically in the splenic surgical resection specimen and showed mucoid change in the media. In three cases of dissecting aortic aneurysm in which postmortem histology was performed, one confirmed the features of Marfan's syndrome but the other two made no comment and the description of the autopsy was inadequate for confirmation. In the one case of dissection of the coronary artery, histology was limited to this site and it was not possible to assess widespread vascular disease. In a further case, of massive retroperitoneal bleeding, death was assumed to be due to rupture of an aneurysm which could not be identified at autopsy.

Varicella infection

Four Indirect deaths were attributed to varicella infection but there was no autopsy in two. In the remaining two, there was inadequate histology and no comment on viral inclusions in one, and no histology in the second.

Discussion

As the number of maternal deaths diminishes it becomes more important that the 'hard core' of deaths each triennium is carefully reviewed so that an accurate picture of events is built up. The autopsy and its associated investigations form an important part of this review. It must therefore be seen as a disappointment that such a high proportion of inadequate autopsies as are here analysed form the basis of the pathological assessment. The attention of coroners and procurators fiscal must be drawn to the fundamental importance of the Confidential Enquiries. It is not only that authority should be granted to perform an autopsy but that these maternal autopsies should be carried out by pathologists with sufficient time, experience and competence to undertake a complete examination and to deliver a fully informative report. Pathologists appropriate for this task should agree to remain as assessors only so long as they can meet these criteria.

The case notes should always be supplied with the request for an autopsy from whatever source. Ideally the obstetrician and anaesthetist should attend or at least be contacted personally so that the attention of the pathologist may be drawn to those points of particular clinical importance for more detailed examination.

In some places, pathologists undertaking autopsies at the request of coroners/procurators fiscal have been reluctant to retain tissue for histological examination unless so instructed. Where coroners/procurators fiscal recognise the necessity of histological examination to establish a cause of death, for example amniotic fluid embolism, such instruction is usually given. However, in all cases of Direct and Indirect maternal death a more detailed histological examination is required and pathologists should discuss this with coroners/procurators fiscal and, if necessary with their Health Authorities/Boards, so that satisfactory arrangements can be implemented.

The care and attention given to this work by some pathologists highlights the deficiencies in others. Although it is the deficiencies that have been emphasised in this report, by the same measure it must be recorded that many autopsies are of the highest standard. These include detailed descriptions and measurements of the anatomical findings. Various appropriate special techniques are used, such as postmortem angiography, enzyme staining of myocardium for the detection and localisation of ischaemia, microbiological and toxicological analysis, often involving multiple sites, and extensive microscopy including immunohistology and electron microscopy.

The autopsy assessment should be extended to include the placenta, stillborn fetus, hysterectomy specimen or other resection specimen such as an aneurysm. Where the experience of any one pathologist is insufficient, the skills of another should be called upon. This applies particularly to neuropathology, cardiac pathology and obstetric pathology. Such collaboration, is regrettably still too uncommon. Blocks of all histology taken should be supplied to the appropriate pathology assessor in all cases. This is of importance not only for their proper assessment but also for building up a library of sufficient range for postgraduate training. Assessors should be encouraged to hold seminars in their Region every three years which would profitably be linked to publication of the report.

The greatest deficiencies remain in the poor quality of anatomical descriptions and in the failure to take and to report on tissue for microscopy. Many preprinted report forms are inappropriate for recording details such as are required in maternal deaths. Subjective statements of size and weight are much less informative than definitive measurements, accurately taken. Microscopy should be sufficiently extensive to ensure that systemic lesions which may not be macroscopically visible have a reasonable chance of being detected. This applies especially to the lesions of hypertension and amniotic fluid embolism.

With the advent of medical audit it will behove all pathologists to review their autopsy reporting, particularly of maternal deaths where the report is of such critical importance.

Conclusion

This chapter emphasises the need for better communication between all those concerned in the clinical care and investigation of these patients. In particular, pathologists need to ascertain what evidence is required in the investigation of maternal deaths and ensure that the necessary resources are made available to provide it. The central role of expert panels of pathologists needs to be emphasised and coroners reminded of them so that greater use may be made of their experience. Pathologists undertaking this work must liaise closely with the Regional/National pathology assessors.

Table 16.1 *Subjective assessment of the adequacy of autopsies in Direct maternal deaths 1985–87, United Kingdom.*

Chapter	Total Deaths	Autopsies			Histology	
		None	Satis	Unsatis	Satis	Unsat/ no record
Hypertensive disorders of pregnancy	27	2	18	7	13	12
Antepartum and postpartum haemorrhage	10	1	8	1	4	5
Thrombosis and thromboembolism						
Pulmonary embolism	29	4	17	8	12	13
Cerebral venous thrombosis	2	1	1	0	0	1
Cerebral arterial thrombosis	1	0	1	0	1	0
Amniotic fluid embolism	9	0	8	1	9	0
Early pregnancy deaths						
Ectopic pregnancy	16	1	11	4	5	10
Abortion	6	1	3	2	2	3
Genital tract sepsis	6	0	4	2	4	2
Genital tract trauma	6	1	4	1	4	1
Deaths associated with anaesthesia	6	1	3	2	3	2
Other Direct deaths	20	1	12	7	11	8
Cardiac disease associated with pregnancy	1	0	1	0	1	0
Late deaths	6	1	2	3	0	5
Totals	145	14	93	38	69	62

Note: Histology reports listed as unsat/no record do not include patients on whom an autopsy was not performed.

Table 16.2 *Subjective assessment of the adequacy of autopsies in Indirect maternal deaths 1985–87, United Kingdom.*

Chapter	Total Deaths	Autopsies			Histology	
		None	Satis	Unsatis	Satis	Unsatis/ no record
Infectious diseases	10	4	6	0	2	4
Neoplastic diseases	4	0	2	2	0	4
Endocrine and metabolic disorders and immune disorders	5	2	1	2	3	0
Diseases of the central nervous system	19	8	8	3	7	4
Diseases of the circulatory system						
Aneurysms and miscellaneous	8	0	8	0	5	3
Cardiac disease	22	3	16	3	13	6
Other Indirect deaths	7	1	3	3	4	2
Sudden unnatural deaths	9	3	2	4	1	5
Late deaths	10	4	5	1	5	1
Totals	94	25	51	18	40	29

Note: Histology reports listed as unsat/no record do not include patients on whom an autopsy was not performed. The figures do not include 26 Fortuitous deaths.

CHAPTER 17

Recommendations

The purpose of this chapter is to highlight the principal lessons which can be learnt from a review of the major causes of maternal death.

The continued downward trend of maternal mortality has been maintained in this triennium. There were 139 Direct deaths as compared with 163 in the United Kingdom in 1982–84, a reduction of 15%, and this must be regarded as evidence of improved maternity care. However it is clear from the persistence of substandard care in the majority of deaths that it is possible to achieve a further reduction in the number of women dying during pregnancy.

Hypertensive disorders of pregnancy

1. All those involved in providing care for a woman with moderate or severe pre-eclampsia should be reminded that there are serious risks for the mother as well as the fetus.

2. An expert team capable of advising or accepting for care any woman with severe pre-eclampsia or eclampsia should be established in every Region. The team should consist of obstetricians, physicians, anaesthetists and midwives who are selected for their interest and experience in dealing with these conditions.

3. Women with severe pre-eclampsia or eclampsia are best cared for in a centralised high-dependency area (see recommendation 3a for 'Deaths associated with anaesthesia'. If such an area is not available, consideration should be given to providing care in an intensive care unit (ICU), even if it means transfer to another hospital.

Antepartum and postpartum haemorrhage

1. All high risk patients likely to require operative delivery, especially those with religious objections to the use of blood and blood products, should be booked for delivery in hospitals with facilities for high dependency or intensive care.

2. Any woman admitted with recurrent or a moderately severe episode of vaginal bleeding, even if not heavy, should be seen as soon as possible by the most senior obstetrician in the duty team.

3. Any woman who has severe uncontrolled obstetric haemorrhage is at

considerable risk until the bleeding has been stopped. All available expertise from haematologists, obstetricians and anaesthetists must be mobilised
to deal with the problem at an early stage.

4. An agreed protocol for dealing with severe haemorrhage (see Annexe to
Chapter 3) should be available in every maternity unit.

Thrombosis and thromboembolism

1. Whenever the diagnosis has been made or there is a strong suspicion
that thromboembolism is present, serious consideration should be given to
treatment for the rest of pregnancy with an anticoagulant such as heparin.
It has to be remembered that more than half the deaths from thromboembolism occurred before 32 weeks of pregnancy.

2. All available methods to establish the diagnosis of thromboembolism
should be used. Radioactive isotopes for this purpose are not contraindicated in the latter half of pregnancy.

Amniotic fluid embolism

Amniotic fluid embolism must always be considered as a cause of sudden
collapse or death in labour or shortly thereafter. In such cases a careful
autopsy should always be performed by a pathologist who specifically
looks for evidence of amniotic fluid embolism in the lungs, and in the
uterus when a hysterectomy has been done prior to death.

Early pregnancy deaths (including abortion)

The following investigations are recommended for any woman suspected
of having an ectopic pregnancy:−

1. Diagnosis of pregnancy using the highly sensitive beta-hCG test
which should be available in general practitioner surgeries, Accident
and Emergency departments and gynaecology wards.

2. An ultrasound scan should be done by an experienced ultrasono-
grapher to determine whether or not there is a pregnancy present and
if it is intrauterine.

3. If there is any doubt of the diagnosis of ectopic pregnancy, especially
if a woman of reproductive age has persisting unexplained lower
abdominal pain, a laparoscopy should be done.

4. The possibility of ectopic pregnancy should be considered in the
reproductive years of life, even if potentially effective methods of contraception are being used, in the presence of lower abdominal pain with
or without associated vaginal bleeding.

Genital tract sepsis

1. Acute genital tract sepsis should be borne in mind as a cause of profound persisting shock and should be treated with broad spectrum antibiotics even in the absence of the classical signs of bacteraemia.

2. A suitable broad-spectrum combination of antibiotics should be used which covers anaerobes and streptococci eg amoxycillin, metronidazole and gentamicin.

3. Bacteriological advice should be obtained at an early stage in all cases of acute genital tract sepsis.

Genital tract trauma

1. The possibility that oxytocics can cause uterine hyperstimulation, or even uterine rupture, should never be forgotten. It needs re-emphasis that, when *Syntocinon* or prostaglandins are used, uterine activity should be monitored continuously.

2. Difficult vaginal operative delivery has been replaced, by and large, by Caesarean section. A consultant should be called at an early stage if a junior obstetrician experiences any difficulty in delivery of a baby by forceps or the ventouse.

Deaths associated with anaesthesia

1. It is essential that a rapid carbon dioxide analyser, pulse oximeter and other appropriate monitoring equipment should be available in any part of the maternity unit where an anaesthetic may be given. Measures must be taken to confirm the correct position of a tracheal tube after every intubation. A procedure for dealing with a failed intubation must be agreed by the anaesthetists and made available to anaesthetists working in the maternity unit.

2. An anaesthetist should be involved early in the management of cases of severe pre-eclampsia, even if operative delivery is not planned, to assist with analgesia, sedation, anti-hypertensive therapy and monitoring. All anaesthetists should be trained in the management of pre-eclampsia and eclampsia.

3. All maternity units where anaesthetics are regularly given should have a postoperative recovery area.

   a. Large maternity units should provide a centralised high-dependency care area, with trained staff and appropriate monitoring equipment, to improve the care of acutely ill patients.

   b. Small maternity units should be capable of providing high-dependency care on an occasional basis within the recovery area.

4. Invasive cardiovascular monitoring should be used when clinically indicated in high risk obstetric patients.

5. Early identification, consultation and planning between obstetricians and anaesthetists is required in the high risk patient. A method of 'flagging' the case notes of patients likely to cause a problem for the anaesthetist should be considered.

6. The availability of consultant anaesthetists, skilled anaesthetic assistants and essential monitoring equipment must be ensured.

Other Direct deaths

1. Deaths continue to occur in women where the cause of antecedent illness is not obvious. Consultation with other specialists at any stage of an unexplained illness inevitably improves the possibility of making a correct diagnosis and instituting appropriate treatment.

2. Whenever a pregnant woman dies unexpectedly it is essential that every effort is made to determine the diagnosis by autopsy. It is the responsibility of the consultant obstetrician concerned to ensure that, if possible, the opinion of an expert obstetric pathologist is available at the autopsy. When permission for an autopsy is not given by the relatives, the possibility of using diagnostic techniques such as liver sampling should be discussed with the relatives.

Cardiac disease associated with pregnancy

1. Pregnant women with cardiac disease should be seen regularly through pregnancy jointly by a cardiologist and obstetrician (unless there is a combined clinic). It is best for one obstetrician to be designated as responsible for the care of all women coming to that maternity unit with cardiac disease.

2. All maternity units should be able to provide emergency cardiac care. If this is not readily available during the antenatal period consideration should be given to transferring serious cases to a maternity unit where such care is available.

3. Every effort should be made to explain the gravity of risks to women with potentially lethal cardiac conditions so that they may be dissuaded from becoming pregnant. Termination of pregnancy may be a better option to recommend than allowing the pregnancy to continue.

4. Intensive care during labour of pregnant women with serious cardiac disease should extend into the postpartum period.

Caesarean section

1. Maternity care is a 24-hour activity and attention must be paid at all

times, night and day, to ensure that the levels of medical and midwifery staffing are adequate to cope with the acute emergencies that often attend Caesarean section. This is particularly relevant to 'split site' units where gynaecology is practised elsewhere.

2. Undue responsibility should not be placed on junior staff, in particular those who are acting up in a more senior post, by expecting them to do an operation beyond the limit of their surgical expertise. It should be recognised that locum doctors and agency midwives must be supervised at all times because the unfamiliar surroundings in which they work put them at greater professional risk.

3. Caesarean section is made more hazardous by lack of adequate facilities. It is essential that an operating theatre is available on every maternity unit to avoid the unavoidable delay that arises when women requiring emergency Caesarean section have to be transferred to theatres elsewhere. Adequate facilities for all forms of resuscitation must be available on site. In particular there should be a postoperative recovery area (see recommendation 3a for 'Deaths associated with anaesthesia', page 146) with equipment for cardiopulmonary resuscitation and blood for transfusion. These recommendations are particularly relevant to maternity units which are separated from a main hospital.

4. Management protocols for resuscitation should always be readily available for every maternity unit.

Pathology

1. Maternal autopsies must be carried out by experienced and competent pathologists who are aware of what needs to be looked for[1] and who give sufficient time to ensure that a thorough examination is carried out. A full and informative report should be provided.

2. The case notes should always be supplied for the pathologist performing the autopsy. The relevant consultants responsible for the clinical care of the deceased should attend the autopsy.

3. Pathologists responsible for autopsies on pregnant women who die should be prepared to carry out the agreed requirements of the enquiry at all times.

4. The attention of coroners and procurators fiscal must be drawn to the importance of meeting the requirements of the Confidential Enquiry into Maternal Deaths. Pathologists undertaking an autopsy at the request of a coroner or procurator fiscal should obtain permission from him to retain tissues such as sample material or amniotic fluid for further detailed examination as required.

5. The autopsy should include the placenta, fetus, and hysterectomy specimen or other tissue removed before death. If a specialised opinion on neuro-, cardiac or obstetric pathology is required, the pathologist should

obtain this advice either from available colleagues or through the appropriate pathology assessor.

6. Regional or National pathology assessors should be encouraged to hold seminars at least every three years. This might profitably take place at the time of publication of the Report.

General recommendations

1. Every consultant maternity unit should have a consultant obstetrician and consultant anaesthetist readily available whose main priority during the period of duty is to oversee the labour ward. The management of many obstetric emergencies requires experience that is only available at consultant level.

2. Any woman with a serious complication(s) of pregnancy must be transferred to a consultant maternity unit with appropriate facilities, including transport, to deal with this complication before her or her baby's life is threatened.

Examples of such complications are worsening pre-eclampsia, preterm labour, and any serious medical or obstetric complication of pregnancy.

3. Split site units where obstetrics and gynaecology are separated are wasteful of staff and facilities, and are potentially dangerous. Isolated units should be moved as soon as possible to part of a general hospital.

4. General practitioners who carry out antenatal care with or without intra-partum care must maintain their skills to keep abreast of changes in practice. Health Authorities should ensure that educational opportunities are available to ensure that this happens. All general practitioners offering maternity services should take part in regular educational activities as recommended by the RCOG/RCGP report (1981)[2].

5. All maternity units should have an assured supply of blood and blood substitutes for administration in any obstetric emergency that may arise, as is required for places approved for termination of pregnancy under the Abortion Act. (See Annex to Chapter 6. Page 62)

Conclusions

There can be no room for complacency despite the fact that it has been shown that the maternal death rate in England and Wales falls by half each decade. Without constant attention to detail and updating of clinical knowledge, the unexpected emergency, which cannot be managed or controlled properly, will inevitably occur. The majority of maternal deaths are still associated with a high degree of substandard care. This cannot be solely explained by deficiency in the provision of facilities, since a major factor in many instances was the level of seniority and experience of those involved. Future planning of the maternity services must therefore allow

149

for a greater involvement of consultants during pregnancy and labour.

The failure to appreciate the severity of a potential complication was a reflection of either inexperience or the decreasing frequency of its occurrence and often both. For whatever reason, it lead to the situation where 'too little too late' was a recurring theme in many of the deaths. The lessons from previous reports obviously take time to generate sufficient attention to produce a marked improvement in standards.

As individual complications become rarer standards have to be raised to detect potential problems at the earliest stage. Whilst pregnancy is a physiological process, it is not without its inherent risk. As advances occur in all disciplines, and defects or diseases are corrected to allow patients to lead a normal life, the inevitable changes associated with pregnancy have to be appreciated by all those concerned, including the woman herself.

The care of a woman during pregnancy and labour has a considerable influence on the generations of tomorrow and therefore deserves greater priority for limited medical resources and staffing. The potential shortage of personnel, medical, midwifery and nursing, over the next decade or two will undoubtedly pose a great challenge and an inevitable reappraisal of the maternity services in the United Kingdom. With foresight, planning and management this should reduce not only maternal mortality but also maternal morbidity.

References

1 Rushton D L, Dawson I M P. The Maternal autopsy. *J Clin Pathol* 1982; 35: 909–921.
2 Feroze R M. Report on training for obstetrics and gynaecology for General Practitioners; report of a Joint Working Group of the RCOG and RCGP. London: Chameleon Press, 1982. Chairman: Mr R M Feroze.

APPENDIX A

Method of the enquiry 1985–87

1. England and Wales

In the case of a known or suspected maternal death, an enquiry was initiated in England by the District Medical Officer (DMO) (now Director of Public Health), or in Wales by the Chief Administrative Medical Officer (CAMO) (now Director of Public Health Medicine/CAMO), of the District in which the woman was usually resident. An enquiry form (MCW97) was sent to general practitioners, midwives, health visitors, consultant obstetricians and any other relevant staff who had been concerned with the care of the woman.

When all the information about the death had been collected the DMO forwarded the form to the appropriate Regional obstetric assessor in England, or the CAMO to the Welsh obstetric assessor. The Regional or Welsh anaesthetic assessors reviewed all cases who had received an anaesthetic. Every possible attempt was made to obtain full details of any postmortem examinations and these were reviewed by the Regional or Welsh pathology assessors. The assessors added their comments and opinions regarding the cause or causes of death.

The MCW97 form was then sent to the Chief Medical Officer of the Department of Health or the Chief Medical Officer of Wales. The Central assessors in obstetrics and gynaecology, anaesthetics and histopathology then reviewed all available recorded facts about each case and assessed the many factors that may have led to death.

2. Scotland

In Scotland, the system of enquiry is similar. However one panel of assessors deals with all cases. Each obstetric assessor is responsible for the geographical area which includes more than one Health Board; there are two anaesthetic assessors each of whom comments on anaesthetic aspects of cases from one half of the country; and one pathology assessor. The allocation of cases to diagnostic category is undertaken by the full panel of assessors each year.

On receipt in the Scottish Home and Health Department (SHHD) of a certificate of maternal death from the General Registrar's Office (Scotland) an enquiry form (MD1) was sent to the Chief Administrative Medical Officer (CAMO) of the Health Board of residence of the woman concerned. As in England and Wales, the CAMO took responsibility for organising completion of the MC1 form by all professional staff involved in caring for

151

the woman. When this was achieved he passed the form to the appropriate obstetric assessor who determined whether further data were required before the case was submitted for discussion and classification to the full panel of assessors. In cases where an anaesthetic had been given or a postmortem or pathological investigation undertaken he passed the form to the appropriate anaesthetic or pathology assessor for their comments. He then returned the form to the Enquiry Co-ordinator (a Senior Medical Officer) at SHHD, who retained it from that time until it had been fully considered, classified and used for preparation of the report. At all times each form was held under conditions of strict confidentiality and was anonymised before being provided to assessors compiling the report.

Additional information was obtained from statistics collected and analysed by the Information and Statistics Division of the Scottish Health Service Common Services Agency. This is available from routine hospital discharge data collected by general and maternity hospitals. The coverage by Form SMR2, the maternal discharge summary, is now almost universal at 98% of registered births. General practitioners and hospital and community medical and nursing staff assisted in ensuring that deaths occurring at home were included in the enquiry.

3. *Northern Ireland*

Deaths due to or associated with pregnancy, childbirth or abortion were reported to the Chief Administrative Medical Officer (CAMO) of the appropriate Health and Social Services Board, who initiated completion of the maternal death form (MCW2 Rev. 2, 1981) by those involved in the care of the patient. All those providing information understood that this would be treated in strict confidence. On completion forms were sent to the Department of Health and Social Services. The Obstetric Assessor reviewed each case and where an anaesthetic had been given it was passed to the Anaesthetic Assessor. The details of postmortem examinations were scrutinised by the Pathology Assessor. The Assessors were asked to consider the report, to give their views of classification and indicate whether avoidable factors were present.

4. *Editorial Board*

The four countries collected their individual cases and these were assessed by their assessors as described above. When the chapters of the report were being written, the authors, all members of the Editorial Board, (see page ii) included relevant cases from all four countries and agreed with their colleagues the final classification of the main causes of death, and the allocation to substandard care (see page x).

Strict confidentiality is observed at all stages of the enquiry, and the identity of the patient is erased from all forms, so that the opinions of the assessors cannot be related to a named individual. After preparation of the report all the maternal death forms are destroyed.

5. *Definitions*

Cause of death

A single *main* cause of death has been allotted and subsequently classified according to the International Classification of Diseases, Injuries and causes of Death — ninth revision (ICD9) (See Tables A1, A2 and A3). This was not necessarily the immediate cause of death. Although deaths are assigned to one main cause, they may be referred to in other chapters; thus a death assigned to hypertensive disorder of pregnancy, in which haemorrhage and anaesthesia also played a part, may be discussed in all three chapters.

Classification of maternal death

There is an international agreement to subdivide causes of obstetric deaths into *Direct* and *Indirect*. ICD9 defines *Direct* obstetric deaths as 'those resulting from obstetric complications of the pregnant state (Pregnancy, labour and puerperium), from interventions, omissions, incorrect treatment, or from a chain of events resulting from any of the above'. *Indirect* deaths are defined as 'those resulting from previous existing disease, or disease that developed during pregnancy and which was not due to direct obstetric causes, but which was aggravated by the physiologic effects of pregnancy'. Only those deaths from other causes which happen to occur in pregnancy or the puerperium are excluded from maternal mortality as internationally defined. For the purpose of the enquiry, these are defined as *Fortuitous* deaths.

Conceptions and pregnancies

It is now customary for the Office of Population Censuses and Surveys (OPCS) to publish annual estimates of conceptions. This is a count of maternities and legal terminations to mothers resident in England and Wales, adjusted to take account of the gestation recorded on the abortion notification.

An alternative denominator has been used in past Reports for the computation of rates where the numerator includes deaths occurring early in pregnancy. These included abortions, ectopic pregnancies and anaesthesia. The number of pregnancies was estimated by adding the number of conceptions (see above) to the estimated number of ectopic pregnancies and spontaneous abortions admitted to NHS hospitals. In the absence of hospital episode statistics it has not been possible in this report to estimate the number of pregnancies in the same way (See Foreword p. ix).

'Late' deaths

ICD9 defines a maternal death as 'the death of a woman while pregnant or within 42 days of termination of pregnancy, from any cause related to or aggravated by the pregnancy or its management, but not from accidental or incidental causes.'. This is in accord with the definition developed by the International Federation of Gynaecology and Obstetrics (FIGO).

In the Confidential Enquiry, however, some deaths have also been included if they occurred between 43 days and one year after delivery or abortion. These 'Late' deaths are considered separately in Chapter 15.

Maternities

In this report deaths are usually related to the number of *maternities*. This is a count of the numbers of mothers *delivered* as distinct from the number of *babies* born; which, of course, includes twins and other multiple births.

Parity

Parity is defined here as the number of previous pregnancies of 28 weeks gestation or more (regardless of the outcome of the pregnancy) plus the present pregnancy, whatever the duration. Birth Registration information about previous births is confined to legally registrable births within marriage so that the construction of a parity distribution of all maternities (Appendix Table A6) required the allocation of births outside marriage by parity plus some reallocation of births within marriage. This has been done in England and Wales by using statistics from the General Household Survey, a sample enquiry conducted each year by the Social Survey Division of OPCS currently covering people in approximately ten thousand private households (one in two thousand of the population). It was not possible to do similar estimates for Scotland and Northern Ireland, and date presented by parity have been dropped from the individual cause of death chapters. (See Foreword p. x).

Substandard Care

For definition, see Foreword page x.

Table A1 *Direct maternal deaths. Deaths due to or associated with pregnancy and childbirth, United Kingdom, 1985–87.*

ICD No.	Cause of death	Assigned code	OPCS code	Late deaths Assigned code	OPCS code
I.	*Infectious and parasitic diseases*				
038	Septicaemia	—	1	—	—
II.	*Neoplasms*				
181	Malignant neoplasm of placenta	—	—	2	2
IV.	*Diseases of blood and blood forming organs*				
286	Coagulation defects	—	2	—	—
VII.	*Diseases of the circulatory system*				
415	Acute pulmonary heart disease	—	1	—	—
424	Other diseases of the endocardium	—	1	—	—
425	Cardiomyopathy	—	1	—	—
427	Cardiac dysrhythmias	—	1	—	—
431	Intracerebral haemorrhage	—	1	—	—
434	Occlusion of cerebral arteries	—	1	—	—
441	Aortic aneurysm	—	1	—	—
453	Other venous embolism and thrombosis	—	5	—	—
459	Other disorders of circulatory system	—	1	—	—
VIII.	*Diseases of the respiratory system*				
493	Asthma	—	1	—	—
518	Other diseases of the lung	—	3	—	—
IX.	*Diseases of the digestive system*				
571	Chronic liver disease and cirrhosis	—	1	—	—
577	Diseases of pancreas	—	1	—	—

ICD No.	Cause of death	Assigned code	OPCS code	Late deaths Assigned code	Late deaths OPCS code
X.	*Diseases of the genitourinary system*				
590	Infections of the kidney	—	1	—	—
621	Disorders of uterus, not elsewhere classified	—	2	—	—
XI.	*Complications of pregnancy, childbirth and the puerperium*				
633	Ectopic pregnancy	15	14	—	—
634	Spontaneous abortion	2	2	—	—
635	Legally induced abortion	1	2	—	—
637	Unspecified abortion	2	—	—	—
639	Complications following abortion and ectopic and molar pregnancies	3	—	—	—
641	Antepartum haemorrhage, abruptio placentae and placenta praevia	4	4	—	—
642	Hypertension complicating pregnancy, childbirth and the puerperium	27	18	—	—
646	Other complications of pregnancy, not elsewhere classified	12	6	—	—
647	Infective and parasitic conditions in the mother classifiable elsewhere but complicating pregnancy, childbirth and the puerperium	2	—	—	—
648	Other current conditions in the mother classifiable elsewhere but complicating pregnancy, childbirth and the puerperium	—	2	—	—
654	Abnormality of organs and soft tissues of pelvis	—	1	—	—
657	Polyhydramnios	—	1	—	—
658	Other problems associated with amniotic cavity and membranes	—	1	—	—
662	Long labour	—	—	—	1
663	Umbilical cord complications	—	1	—	—
665	Other obstetrical trauma	6	5	—	—
666	Postpartum haemorrhage	6	6	—	—
667	Retained placenta or membranes, without haemorrhage	—	1	—	—
668	Complications of the administration of anaesthetic or other sedation in labour and delivery	6	1	2	—
669	Other complications of labour and delivery not elsewhere classified	1	6	—	1
670	Major puerperal infection	4	2	1	—
671	Venous complications in pregnancy and the puerperium	3	15	—	1
673	Obstetrical pulmonary embolism	39	14	1	—
674	Other and unspecified complications of the puerperium, not elsewhere classified	6	3	—	1
XVII.	*Injury and poisoning*				
933	Foreign body in pharynx and larynx	—	1	—	—
934	Foreign body in trachea, bronchus and lung	—	1	—	—
994	Effects of other external causes	—	1	—	—
997	Complications affecting specified body systems, not elsewhere classified	—	1	—	—
Total		139	134*	6	6

* There are 5 cases where OPCS codes have not been notified.

Table A2 *Indirect maternal deaths, United Kingdom, 1985–87.*

ICD No.	Cause of death	Assigned code	OPCS code	Late deaths Assigned code	Late deaths OPCS code
I.	*Infectious and parasitic diseases*				
013	Tuberculosis of meninges and central nervous system	—	1	—	—
034	Streptococcal sore throat and scarlatina	—	1	—	—
052	Chickenpox	—	1	—	—
070	Viral hepatitis	—	1	—	—
II.	*Neoplasms*				
183	Malignant neoplasm of ovary and other uterine adnexa	—	1	—	—
202	Other malignant neoplasm of lymphoid and histiocytic tissue	—	1	—	—
227	Benign neoplasm of other endocrine glands and related structures	—	2	—	—
239	Neoplasm of unspecified nature	—	2	—	—
IV.	*Diseases of blood and blood forming organs*				
282	Hereditary haemolytic anaemias	—	1	—	—
285	Other and unspecified anaemias	—	1	—	—
V.	*Mental disorders*				
305	Nondependent abuse of drugs	—	2	—	—
VI.	*Diseases of the nervous system and sense organs*				
324	Intracranial and intraspinal abscess	—	1	—	—
345	Epilepsy	—	3	—	—
VII.	*Diseases of the circulatory system*				
394	Diseases of mitral valve	—	1	—	—
410	Acute myocardial infarction	—	1	—	—
414	Other forms of chronic ischaemic heart disease	—	1	—	—
416	Chronic pulmonary heart disease	—	1	—	—
420	Acute pericarditis	—	1	—	—
421	Acute and subacute endocarditis	—	1	—	—
430	Subarachnoid haemorrhage	—	6	—	1
431	Intracerebral haemorrhage	—	1	—	—
434	Occlusion of cerebral arteries	—	1	—	—
441	Aortic aneurysm	—	2	—	—
442	Other aneurysm	—	3	—	—
448	Diseases of capillaries	—	1	—	—
459	Other disorders of circulatory system	—	1	—	—
VIII.	*Diseases of the respiratory system*				
486	Pneumonia, organism unspecified	—	—	—	1
493	Asthma	—	1	—	—
IX.	*Diseases of the digestive system*				
560	Intestinal obstruction without mention of hernia	—	1	—	—
570	Acute and subacute necrosis of liver	—	—	—	1
X.	*Diseases of genitourinary system*				
590	Infections of kidney	—	1	—	—

Table A2—*continued*

ICD No.	Cause of death	Assigned code	OPCS code	Late deaths Assigned code	Late deaths OPCS code
XI.	*Complications of pregnancy, childbirth and the puerperium*				
630	Hydatidiform mole	—	1	—	—
634	Spontaneous abortion	—	1	—	—
641	Antepartum haemorrhage, abruptio placentae, and placenta praevia	—	1	—	—
642	Hypertension complicating pregnancy, childbirth and the puerperium	—	2	—	—
646	Other complications of pregnancy, not elsewhere classified	3	3	—	—
647	Infective and parasitic conditions in the mother classifiable elsewhere, but complicating pregnancy, childbirth and the puerperium:				
.3	Tuberculosis	1	—	—	—
.6	Other viral diseases	5	3	—	—
.8	Other specified infective and parasitic diseases	4	—	—	—
648	Other current conditions in the mother classifiable elsewhere, but complicating pregnancy, childbirth and the puerperium:				
.0	Diabetes mellitus	2	—	—	—
.2	Anaemia	1	1	—	—
.3	Drug dependence	1	—	—	—
.4	Mental disorders	9	1	3	—
.5	Congenital cardiovascular disorders	10	2	—	—
.6	Other cardiovascular diseases	20	9	1	—
.8	Abnormal glucose tolerance	—	1	—	—
.9	Other	13	—	2	—
669	Other complications of labour and delivery, not elsewhere classified	—	—	—	1
670	Major puerperal infection	—	—	1	1
673	Obstetrical pulmonary embolism	—	1	—	—
674	Other and unspecified complications of the puerperium, not elsewhere classified	15	4	2	—
XIV.	*Congenital anomalies*				
746	Other congenital abnormalities of the heart	—	1	—	—
759	Other and unspecified congenital anomalies	—	2	—	—
XVI.	*Symptoms, signs and ill-defined conditions*				
799	Other ill-defined and unknown causes of morbidity and mortality	—	1	—	—
XVII.	*Injury and poisoning*				
851	Cerebral laceration and contusion	—	1	—	—
952	Spinal cord lesion without evidence of spinal bone injury	—	1	—	—
965	Poisoning by analgesics, antipyretics and antirheumatics	—	—	1	1
994	Effects of other external causes	—	1	1	2
	External causes of injury and poisoning				
E890	Conflagration in private dwelling	—	1	—	—
E910	Accidental drowning and submersion	—	1	—	—
E950	Suicide and self inflicted poisoning by solid or liquid substance	—	1	—	—
E958	Suicide and self inflicted injury by other and unspecified means	—	1	—	—
Total		84	83*	8	8

* There is 1 case of Indirect death where OPCS code has not been notified.

Table A3 *Fortuitous maternal deaths, United Kingdom, 1985–87.*

ICD No.	Cause of death	Assigned code	OPCS code	Late deaths Assigned code	Late deaths OPCS code
I.	*Infectious and parasitic diseases*				
049	Other non-arthropod-borne viral diseases of central nervous system	1	1	—	—
070	Viral hepatitis	1	1	—	—
II.	*Neoplasms*				
151	Malignant neoplasm of stomach	1	—	—	—
154	Malignant neoplasm of rectum, rectosigmoid junction and anus	1	1	—	—
172	Malignant melanoma of skin	1	1	—	—
174	Malignant neoplasm of female breast	1	1	1	1
191	Malignant neoplasm of brain	3	1	—	—
199	Malignant neoplasm without specification of site	—	1	—	—
202	Other malignant neoplasm of lymphoid and histiocytic tissue	1	—	—	—
205	Myeloid leukaemia	1	1	—	—
206	Monocytic leukaemia	2	1	—	—
225	Benign neoplasm of brain and other parts of nervous system	1	1	—	—
239	Benign neoplasm of other and unspecified sites	—	1	—	—
IV.	*Diseases of blood and blood-forming organs*				
282	Hereditary haemolytic anaemias	—	1	—	—
VI.	*Diseases of the nervous system and the sense organs*				
320	Bacterial meningitis	1	—	—	—
VII.	*Diseases of the circulatory system*				
414	Other forms of chronic ischaemic heart disease	1	1	—	—
421	Acute and subacute endocarditis	1	—	—	—
428	Heart failure	—	1	—	—
VIII.	*Diseases of the respiratory system*				
493	Asthma	4	2	—	—
XI.	*Complications of pregnancy, childbirth and the puerperium*				
648	Other current conditions in the mother classifiable elsewhere but complicating pregnancy, childbirth and the puerperium	—	2	—	—
XVII.	*Injury and poisoning*				
852	Subarachnoid, subdural and extradural haemorrhage following injury	—	1	—	—
947	Burns of internal organs	1	—	—	—
987	Toxic effect of other gases, fumes or vapours	—	1	—	—
	External causes of injury and poisoning				
E812	Other motor vehicle traffic accident involving collision with another motor vehicle	2	2	—	—
E815	Other motor vehicle traffic accident involving collision on the highway	1	1	—	—
E818	Other noncollision motor vehicle traffic accident	—	—	—	1
E819	Motor vehicle traffic accident of unspecified nature	1	—	—	—
Total		26	23*	3	3

* There are 3 cases of Fortuitous deaths where OPCS codes have not been notified.

Table A4 *Number of deaths by age of mother in the Enquiry for England and Wales 1982–84 compared with those included in England and Wales and the UK 1985–87, and the rate per million maternities.*

Number of maternal deaths

Age	England and Wales 1982–84 Direct	Indirect	Fortuitous	England and Wales 1985–87 Direct	Indirect	Fortuitous	United Kingdom 1985–87 Direct	Indirect	Fortuitous
Under 16	—	—	—	—	—	—	—	—	—
16–17	2	1	—	1	—	1	1	—	1
18–19	7	6	4	10	2	4	11	3	5
20–24	27	16	7	21	22	8	24	23	8
25–29	39	19	12	30	14	4	34	19	4
30–34	28	13	5	30	22	2	36	24	3
35–39	27	13	6	25	6	3	28	7	5
40–44	8	3	—	4	6	—	5	6	—
45+	—	—	—	—	1	—	—	2	—
Total	138	71	34	121	73	22	139	84	26

Rate per million maternities

Age	England and Wales 1982–84 Direct	Indirect	Fortuitous	England and Wales 1985–87 Direct	Indirect	Fortuitous	United Kingdom 1985–87 Direct	Indirect	Fortuitous
16–17	54.8*	42.6*	24.4*	64.0*	11.6*	5.8*	62.6*	15.7*	5.2*
20–24	47	27.9	12.2	36.4	38.1	6.9	37.1	35.6	7.7
25–29	60.9	29.7	18.7	43.4	20.3	11.6	43.7	24.4	10.3
30–34	77.4	35.9	13.8	77.1	38.1	10.3	82.3	54.9	9.1
35–39	220.7	106.3	49.1	185.0	44.4	14.8	184.1	46.0	19.7
40–44	482.4	160.6	—	169.3	254.0	127.0	187.7	225.3	187.7
Total	73.3	37.7	18.0	60.9	36.7	11.1	62.3	37.6	11.6

* Rates for ages under 20.

Table A5 *Number of deaths by parity of mother in the Enquiry for England and Wales 1982–84 compared with those included in 1985–87 and the rate per million maternities.*

Number of maternal deaths

Parity	England and Wales 1982–84 Direct	Indirect	Fortuitous	England and Wales 1985–87 Direct	Indirect	Fortuitous	United Kingdom 1985–87 Direct	Indirect	Fortuitous
1	56	26	11	48	28	7	57	30	9
2	32	23	11	26	20	7	28	22	8
3	26	11	3	17	9	1	19	11	2
4	16	7	5	15	8	3	17	10	3
5–9	8	4	3	12	7	4	15	10	4
10+	—	—	—	—	1	—	—	1	—
NS	—	—	1	3	—	—	3	—	—
Total	138	71	34	121	73	22	139	84	26

Rate per million maternities

Parity	England and Wales 1982–84 Direct	Indirect	Fortuitous	England and Wales 1985–87 Direct	Indirect	Fortuitous	United Kingdom 1985–87 Direct	Indirect	Fortuitous
1	73.4	34.1	14.4	60.3	33.8	8.4	60.9	32.0	9.6
2	49.0	35.2	16.8	40.8	30.2	10.6	37.8	29.7	10.8
3	88.8	37.6	10.3	55.6	29.4	3.3	55.5	32.2	5.8
4	149.2	65.3	46.6	130.7	69.7	26.1	133.1	78.3	23.5
5–9	118.7	59.3	44.5	156.7	91.4	52.2	177.4	118.3	47.3
10+	—	—	—	—	—	—	—	—	—
NS	—	—	—	—	—	—	—	—	—
Total	73.3	37.7	18.0	60.9	36.7	11.1	62.3	37.6	11.6

159

Table A6 *True birth order — maternities England and Wales 1970–87, compared with United Kingdom 1985–87*

Years	True birth order*	Total	Age groups					
			Under 20	20–24	25–29	30–34	35–39	40+
1970–87 England & Wales	1	4,735,729	925,232	1,864,638	1,398,604	436,480	95,550	15,225
	2	4,085,370	186,916	1,347,019	1,632,055	718,205	173,614	27,561
	3	1,787,406	18,904	387,569	669,616	512,952	169,839	28,526
	4	681,311	2,260	105,110	242,957	202,545	105,656	22,783
	5+	474,194	146	24,852	122,743	155,628	118,522	52,303
Total		11,764,010	1,133,458	3,729,188	4,065,975	2,025,810	663,181	146,398
1985–87 England & Wales	1	829,439	146,291	302,647	255,530	99,148	22,997	2,826
	2	661,208	22,855	193,706	263,354	136,085	39,801	5,407
	3	305,945	2,253	58,734	108,010	96,440	35,369	5,139
	4	114,745	457	16,855	43,162	31,119	19,337	3,815
	5+	76,577	31	5,369	20,979	26,143	17,620	6,435
Total		1,987,914	171,887	577,311	691,035	388,935	135,124	23,622
1985–87 United Kingdom	1	936,224	163,151	341,550	290,357	112,013	25,972	3,181
	2	741,164	25,566	216,096	295,478	153,798	44,294	5,932
	3	342,111	2,441	64,778	121,852	107,514	39,776	5,750
	4	127,732	471	18,101	47,410	35,409	21,993	4,348
	5+	84,566	34	5,619	22,580	28,821	20,087	7,425
Total		2,231,797	191,663	646,144	777,677	437,555	152,122	26,636

1981 figures are based on a 10% sample for age-group and parity.

* Previous live births regardless of legitimacy. Birth registration figures adjusted using information from the 1970–82 General Household Survey. Adjustment factors derived from the 1979–82 GHS have been applied to convert live births to estimated maternities.

Table A7 *Number of Direct Maternal Deaths included in the Enquiry by age and parity, United Kingdom 1985–87.*

Age (years)	Parity							
	1	2	3	4	5–9	10+	Not stated	All
Under 16	—	—	—	—	—	—	—	—
16–17	1	—	—	—	—	—	—	1
18–19	8	3	—	—	—	—	—	11
20–24	15	6	1	1	1	—	—	24
25–29	13	9	7	1	3	—	1	34
30–34	10	6	7	6	5	—	2	36
35–39	9	4	2	7	6	—	—	28
40–44	1	—	2	2	—	—	—	5
Not stated	—	—	—	—	—	—	—	—
Total	57	28	19	17	15	—	3	139

Table A8 *Rate per 100,000 Maternities of Direct Maternal Deaths included in the Enquiry by age and parity, United Kingdom 1985–87.*

Age (years)	Parity					
	1	2	3	4	5+	All
Under 20	55.2	117.3	—	—	—	62.6
20–24	43.9	27.8	15.4	55.2	178.0	37.1
25–29	44.8	30.5	57.4	21.1	132.9	43.7
30–34	89.3	39.0	65.1	169.5	173.5	82.3
35–39	346.5	90.3	50.3	318.3	298.7	184.1
40+	314.4	—	347.8	460.0	—	187.7
Total	60.9	37.8	55.5	133.1	177.4	62.3

APPENDIX B

Acknowledgements

This report has been made possible by the help and work of the District Medical Officers in England and Chief Administrative Officers in Wales, Scotland and Northern Ireland who initiated case reports and collected the information and the consultant obstetricians, anaesthetists and pathologists, general practitioners and midwives who have supplied the detailed case records and autopsy reports.

Considerable assistance has also been given by procurators fiscal who have supplied copies of reports of autopsies, and by coroners who have supplied autopsy reports and sometimes inquest proceedings to the assessors on request.

The staff of the Medical Statistics Division of the Office of Population Censuses and Surveys in England have worked with the Information and Statistics Division of the Common Services Agency in Scotland and departmental statisticians in Wales and Northern Ireland to prepare the Introduction to the Report, process the statistical data and prepare the Tables and Figures.

The Editorial Board would like to express their thanks to all these people and also in particular to the consultant obstetricians, anaesthetists and pathologists listed below who have acted as regional assessors in England and assessors in Scotland and helped in the preparation of this report.

I. ENGLISH REGIONAL ASSESSORS IN OBSTETRICS

Northern Region	Professor W Dunlop FRCS FRCOG
Yorkshire Region	Mr A G Gordon FRCS FRCOG
Trent Region	Professor J MacVicar MD FRCS FRCOG
East Anglian Region	Mr J A Carron Brown FRCS FRCOG
North West Thames Region	Mr A C Fraser FRCOG
North East Thames Region	Mr G L Bourne FRCS FRCOG (until 31.8.87) Professor H A Brant MD FRCP FRCS FRCOG (from 1.9.87)
South East Thames Region	Mr E D Morris MD FRCS FRCOG
South West Thames Region	Professor G V P Chamberlain MD FRCS FRCOG
Oxford Region	Mr G Mitford Barberton FRCOG
South Western Region	Mr A Howard John FRCS FRCOG (until 31.1.88) Professor G M Stirrat MA MD FRCOG (from 1.2.88)

West Midlands Region:
Sub-Region I   Mr H Oliphant Nicholson FRCS FRCOG (until
                      31.8.87 — whole Region from 1.9.87)
Sub-Region II   Mr K Baker MD FRCOG (until 31.8.87)
North Western Region Mr D W Warrell MD FRCOG (until 31.8.87)
                      Mr P Donnai MA MB BChir FRCOG (from 1.9.87)
Mersey Region   Mrs S H Towers MD FRCOG
Wessex Region   Professor J K Dennis FRCS FRCOG (deceased Dec
                      1989)

II. ENGLISH REGIONAL ANAESTHETIC ASSESSORS

Northern Region   Dr P Stuart MB ChB FFARCS (until 31.8.87)
                      Dr M R Bryson MB BS FFARCS (from 1.9.87)
Yorkshire Region   Dr F R Ellis PhD MB ChB FFARCS
Trent Region   Dr A D G Nicholas MB ChB FFARCS (until
                      31.8.88)
                      Dr J A Caunt MB ChB FFARCS (from 1.9.88)
East Anglian Region   Dr B R Wilkey BM BCh FFARCS
North West Thames
Region   Dr M Morgan MB BS FFARCS
North East Thames
Region   Dr Hilary Howells MB ChB FFARCS
South East Thames
Region   Dr P B Hewitt MB BS FFARCS
South West Thames
Region   Dr H C Churchill Davidson MA MD FFARCS
                      (until 31.8.87)
                      Dr H F Seeley MSc MA MB BS FFARCS (from
                      1.9.87)
Oxford Region   Dr J Edmonds Seal MB BS FFARCS
South Western Region Dr T A Thomas MB ChB FFARCS
West Midlands Region Dr A M Veness MB ChB FFARCS
North Western Region Dr J M Anderton MB ChB FFARCS
Mersey Region   Dr T H L Bryson MB ChB FFARCS
Wessex Region   Dr D J Pearce MB BS FFARCS (until 31.8.87)
                      Professor J Norman PhD MB ChB FFARCS (from
                      1.9.87)

III. ENGLISH REGIONAL ASSESSORS IN PATHOLOGY

Northern Region   Dr E W Walton MD FRCPath
Yorkshire Region   Dr D M Piercy MB ChB FRCPath (until 31.8.87)
                      Dr I N Reid MB ChB MRCPath (from 1.9.87)
Trent Region   Dr A S Hill MA FRCP FRCOG FRCPath
East Anglian Region   Dr P F Roberts MB BS MRCP FRCPath
North West Thames
Region   Dr I A Lampert MB ChB DCP FRCPath
North East Thames
Region   Dr L E McGee MA FRCP FRCPath (until 31.8.87)
                      Dr R G M Letcher MB BS FRCPath (from 1.9.87)

South East Thames Region	Dr M Driver MB BS FRCPath

South East Thames
Region   Dr M Driver MB BS FRCPath
South West Thames
Region   Professor W B Robertson MD FRCPath (until
                       31.8.87)
                       Dr M Hall MB BS FRCPath (from 1.9.87)
Oxford Region   Dr R H Cowdell DM FRCPath (until 31.8.87)
                       Dr W Gray MB BS FRCPath (from 1.9.87)
South Western Region Professor P P Anthony MB BS FRCPath
West Midlands Region Dr D I Rushton MB ChB FRCPath
North Western Region Professor H Fox MD FRCPath
Mersey Region   Dr I W McDicken MD FRCPath
Wessex Region   Dr G H Millward-Sadler BSc MB ChB FRCPath

IV. SCOTTISH ASSESSORS TO THE CEMD NOT SERVING ON THE UK CEMD EDITORIAL BOARD

A. Scottish Assessors who participated in discussion and classification of Scottish cases and commented on draft chapters of the report:

Dr M H Hall MD MBChB FRCOG   )
Dr N B Patel MBChB FRCOG   )
Dr J B Scrimgeour MBChB FRCS FRCOG   ) Obstetric
Dr K S Stewart MD MBChB FRCS FRCOG   )
Dr H P McEwan MD MBChB FRCS FRCOG   )
Dr J Thorburn MBChB FFARCS DObstRCOG   Anaesthetic
Dr E S Gray MBChB MRCPath   Pathology

B. Scottish Assessors who participated in discussion and classification of Scottish cases but had retired before the report was initiated:

Dr J D O Loudon MBChB FRCS FRCOG   )
Dr W P Black MBChB FRCS FRCOG   ) Obstetric
Dr W T Fullerton MBChB FRCOG   )
Dr D D Moir MD FFARCS   Anaesthetic

Printed in the United Kingdom for HMSO
Dd29359   C56   2/91